THE BOY WHO DELIVERED JOY

Marvin Bartlett

The Boy Who Delivered Joy

Published by Gatekeeper Press
2167 Stringtown Rd, Suite 109
Columbus, OH 43123-2989
www.GatekeeperPress.com

ISBN (paperback): 9781642375503
eISBN: 9781642375497

Library of Congress Control Number: 2019949204

Contents

Foreword v

1 The Videotape 1

2 Baby Talk 4

3 Pleasure and Pain 8

4 Diagnosis 13

5 Sixty Days 18

6 Amputation 22

7 Adjustment 28

8 The Cancer Returns 37

9 Sickness in Seattle 41

10 The Dream Factory 49

11 Difficult Journey 54

12 A Kindred Spirit 56

13 Transplant 59

14 The Pink Ladies 62

15 Recovery 64

16 Saying Thanks 71

17 The Silly Season 74

18 "Go, Jarrett, Go" 76

19 After Summer Comes the Fall 80

20 Indian Summer Camp 83

21 Promotion 88

22 An Open Book 90

23 A Perfect Match 94

24 Jarrett Gets an Idea 98

25 My Turn 106

26 A National Audience 111

27 Toyland.. 121

28 Response 125

29 Common Bond 130

30 Metal Head 135

31 Medal Winner 138

32 Chance Meetings... 143

33 Holding Court 152

34 The Banquet and the Bishop 157

35 Oprah 160

36 "You've Got Mail".. 164

37 A Ton of Bricks... 169

38 Something to Say 172

39 Downhill... 176

40 Faith... 185

41 Penny War 193

42 Reflection 198

43 Sequel... 204

44 Some Good Days 210

45 Joy in the Mourning... 215

46 Marching Orders 223

47 Ripples 226

48 No Time to Rest 238

49 To Be Continued 249

Afterword 252

Acknowledgments 255

Links 257

Foreword

When Marvin first asked me if he could write a book about The Joy Cart and me, I thought it was pretty crazy. I couldn't see why anyone would want to read about a kid who's battled cancer most of his life. That doesn't make for very fun reading. But then I thought of all the things I've learned and done because of my cancer.

I decided to let Marvin write this book because I want other people facing tough situations to know that you can get through almost anything if you keep a positive attitude and remember helping others is the best way to help yourself.

There aren't enough words to tell my family, friends, the medical staff and the Jarrett's Joy Cart volunteers and supporters how much I appreciate all they've done. This story would be very different if it weren't for all of you.

—JARRETT MYNEAR
February 2002
Age 12

"In a moment of joy, there is healing."
—Jarrett's Joy Cart motto

1

The Videotape

It was crunch time in the television newsroom, that time of day when you're really up against the deadline. It's the hour when almost all reporters are back from the field, scrambling to type last-second information into their scripts, get videotape edited and phone calls returned. It's a crazy, hectic atmosphere that true journalists love and outside observers find disturbing.

As I made my way through the mayhem to my desk, I wondered if anyone would notice that my eyes were watery. Surely, as big as it felt, that lump in my throat would be visible. I had just viewed a few minutes of videotape of a little boy who was fighting some kind of cancer, and it affected me.

The tape had been shot earlier in the day by a videographer who went alone to the University of Kentucky Children's Hospital. The planned news conference wasn't deemed important enough to require a reporter. It was basketball season in Kentucky, "March Madness," a time when the UK Wildcats were expected to bulldoze their way through all competition and make it to the Final Four. It seemed half our staff was on the road with the team and the other half was scraping up local sidebar stories. If you own a business with "Wildcat" in the name, it may get you a shot on the nightly news in March. If you skip work to watch an afternoon basketball game at a local bar (and thousands do), you might have a camera stuck in your face. The mayor of Lexington declares every day UK is playing a tournament game as "Blue-White Day," meaning you could be chastised by friends and neighbors if you forgot to put on the team colors before you headed out of the house that morning. It's said that basketball is a religion in Kentucky. Our newscasts can sometimes look like a worship service.

That's why the shooter had been instructed to "spray" the news conference. In newsroom lingo, that means "get in and out quickly." We wouldn't have much room for the story in the basketball-heavy show that night.

Little did any of us know that the boy who was the focus of the news conference that day would soon touch us all so deeply.

My assignment as a reporter/anchor was to view the tape, pick a short sound bite, and write a forty-second story for the 5 P.M. newscast. That was my introduction to Jarrett Mynear.

What I saw was a small boy, nine years old at the time, who was more articulate than any child I had ever seen interviewed. Usually when we try to interview someone that age, we get yes-and no-answers and a whole lot of shoulder shrugs, and we hear "I don't know" over and over again. That's O. K. They're little kids. They're not expected to wax poetic.

Yet here was Jarrett speaking in complete and thought-provoking sentences. He had one of those "Owen Meany" type voices. Fans of John Irving will know immediately what I mean. He spoke with a squeak, a sound that commands your attention because of its uniqueness.

The news conference revealed that a new sight would soon be seen around the children's ward. "Jarrett's Joy Cart" would deliver free toys twice a month to every child who was a patient there. And here's where he got me. Jarrett, sitting at a table with his head barely peeking above the microphones, said he knew what it was like to spend most of your life in a hospital.

"Kids get bored and depressed in here," he said. "Some of them never get any visitors."

He said he wanted to deliver toys on a regular schedule to give the patients something to look forward to.

He said it with such sincerity that I knew it wasn't rehearsed. It was the squeaky voice of experience, from someone who should be out on the playground or tossing pebbles in a creek—not someone who should have any idea what it means to spend weeks hooked up to intravenous tubes, facing surgery upon surgery.

As if the words weren't enough to make a direct hit on my soft spot, the pictures sealed the deal. Jarrett had a large bald spot on the back of his head, a circle that marked the spot of one surgery. I later learned that he liked to compare himself to Friar Tuck, and that does indeed best describe his appearance at that time.

After the news conference, the videographer followed The Joy Cart on its inaugural run from room to room, and another surprise showed up on the tape. The boy limped. His right leg was artificial.

With the lump forming in my throat as I viewed the tape, comic relief came at just the right time. As Jarrett pushed the hospital cart loaded down with stuffed animals, games, and puzzles, it got away from him and banged into a wall. Clearly, the microphone picked up his response: "I'm not a very good driver today. I've had too much Coke to drink."

Normally, when writing such a short story about a news conference, I wouldn't even watch the whole tape. But I watched everything we had recorded at the hospital that day and knew right away we had to do more. We weren't doing this story justice. But I banged out the copy for the short segment on the computer, edited the tape, and put it in the mix of things that were about to air.

I watched on a monitor in the newsroom as the story was broadcasted live, and I checked out the reactions of the others around me. These "hardened" journalists who had seen their share of crime, corruption and coroner's cases were touched too, just as I had been. Jarrett had captured everyone's attention in a ten-second sound bite.

I heard my colleagues utter phrases that would probably embarrass most nine-year-old boys.

"He's precious."

"What an angel!"

"How cute!"

The descriptions fit. As we would all soon learn, Jarrett's Joy Cart was destined to do more than deliver toys. It would become a symbol of hope and inspiration to cancer patients everywhere. And the boy behind it, full of Coke or not, would become the best example imaginable of someone who turned life's lemons into lemonade.

2
Baby Talk

Doug Mynear had hoped to have a date when he managed to get two tickets to the University of Kentucky basketball game that January night in 1983. Those tickets should've been easy bait. UK tickets are as precious as jewels in Central Kentucky and more difficult to come by. And the opponent was Southeastern Conference rival Louisiana State University. UK fans loved to come out to heckle Dale Brown, LSU's colorful coach.

But as fate would have it, Doug's date backed out and he had to take his roommate to the game. It turned out to be a wonderful change in plans.

Before the game, a crowd milled around in the Lexington Civic Center just outside Rupp Arena, one of the great shrines of basketball. As Doug and his roommate Mike rode the escalator down to the center's first floor food court, Mike noticed a friend standing in line at a sandwich cart. He went over to greet her and meet her friend, Jennifer Wagner. It was a quick conversation, but Doug knew right away he wouldn't mind talking to Jennifer more.

After the game, the foursome met again at a bar in the Civic Center. Doug's hunches were right. Jennifer was just as nice as she had seemed to be two hours earlier when she had made her first impression.

That was the beginning of a dating relationship that lasted more than a year. They often joked about being the country boy and the city girl. As Jennifer liked to say, she was raised on concrete in Louisville. Doug was a farm boy from Nicholas County, Kentucky. Actually, Doug said he was a country "man." After all, he was thirty years old when they met. She was twenty-six.

The pairing just seemed right. Doug and Jennifer had a big church wedding in Louisville a year and a half after he first spied her from the escalator. Now, he was on another ride, this time going up.

The couple enjoyed each other's company exclusively for nearly four years, taking vacations to Cancun, then Bermuda and Montreal. It seemed neither of them had a care in the world as they hopped on planes, strolled on beaches, and sampled exotic cuisine. They were yuppies with good jobs and the freedom to roam. She worked as a high school special education teacher, meaning she had summers off. He was a civil engineer, helping design things such as drainage systems for highways. Life was good, but after a while, it began to seem incomplete.

When Jennifer found out she was pregnant, she instantly kicked into that mommy-to-be mode. The anticipation of motherhood overwhelmed her. The house was baby-proofed and a nursery was ready months before the due date.

On a Sunday afternoon outing, Jennifer and Doug picked out a name for their baby. They walked a trail at Blue Licks Battlefield State Park, just four miles from Doug's boyhood home. Monuments there list the names of pioneers who tried to defend the region from British soldiers during the American Revolution. Daniel Boone was one of them.

As they scanned one marker, Doug's eyes stopped on the name Jarrett. He remembered that someone in his family tree had had that name two or three generations ago.

"Do you like that name?" he asked Jennifer.

"Very much," she said.

And that was it. It's a good thing they had a boy. Jarrett was the only name they had in mind after that.

Their pioneer namesake arrived April 16, 1989, by Caesarean section after seventeen hours of labor. He was right on time, all eight pounds, eleven ounces of him.

Doug remembers the newness of bringing a baby into the house for the first time.

"We sat his carrier up on the dining room table, and we both just stood there staring at him. Then we looked at each other and said, 'What do we do now?'"

Is anyone ever really prepared for parenthood? Like all new parents, the Mynears became quick experts by on-the-job training. They learned one thing early on. God had blessed them with a happy baby.

Other parents had told them horror stories about babies who cried and screamed all through the night. That was never much of a problem with Jarrett. He usually slept peacefully and when awake, he smiled easily and often.

Everyone likes to brag that they have smart kids, but the Mynears had the evidence to back it up. Jarrett started talking at eight months when he surprised his parents by pointing and asking for a "nana" at breakfast. By ten months, he was forming partial sentences. At one year, he could carry on a conversation.

At his eighteen-month checkup, the pediatrician told the Mynears their son had the vocabulary of a four-year-old.

Doug laughed at how other parents reacted around Jarrett.

"They would have kids who were a year older than he was, and Jarrett could talk rings around them. They'd look at their kids as if to say, 'What's wrong with you?'"

Jarrett's parents said he was attracted to books immediately. They read to him as soon as he was big enough to sit in their laps. For many kids, a bedtime story is a nightly ritual. For Jarrett, being read to was a morning, noon, and night thing. He was always crawling across the floor, dragging a book along beside him, looking for someone to translate the words and pictures to him.

Jarrett was around adults all the time, and that no doubt boosted his development.

In the first year of his life, the infant spent a lot of hours in hospital rooms as Jennifer visited her dying father, a victim of colon cancer.

"My dad was very intolerant of kids and their antics by that time," she said, "but there was no problem bringing Jarrett into his room. Jarrett would sit on the mattress as Dad read to him and gave him rides up and down on the mechanical bed. I think Jarrett picked up a lot of words then."

He also became a baseball fan before the age of one. Doug could hold up a baseball card, and Jarrett would call out the name of the team that claimed the featured player.

"Yankees!"

"Dodgers!"

"Reds!"

That was another trick that impressed his doctors.

When Jarrett could toddle enough to get out of the house, his quests were almost always in search of conversation. A neighbor remembers looking up from beyond her backyard fence one day to see Jarrett, in a diaper, pulling himself up on the deck railing to get a better look at her.

"Holly," he called out in his tiny voice to his neighbor. "You look like you could use some company!"

Holly just shook her head and laughed. The next thing she knew she was engaged in friendly banter with a munchkin.

3

Pleasure and Pain

"Football Weather." That's how our meteorologist summed up such nights, and we all knew what he meant. Anyone going out would need a jacket or sweater, but they wouldn't be too uncomfortable huddled with others in bleachers.

Jennifer and Doug put a coat on their two-and-a-half year old son and went to a game. As a part-time special education teacher at Lexington's Paul Laurence Dunbar High School, Jennifer wanted to show her support for the team. Besides, high school games in Central Kentucky are social gatherings—something to do on a Friday night. The Bulldogs' opponent that night was a state powerhouse, Campbell County. During the game, the couple spent some time actually watching the twenty-two young men go up and down the field. But their attention was divided among friends in the stands, and Jarrett's wide-eyed wonder at everything else going on around him. He watched the mascots, the cheerleaders, and the people who kept coming over to make small talk.

Who won the game? The Mynears' memory is cloudy on that. It's not important because when the final horn sounded, it marked the beginning of turmoil in their lives.

As the threesome stepped out of the bleachers and onto the cold ground, Jarrett looked up at Doug.

"Daddy, carry me. My leg hurts."

That was unusual. Jarrett liked to take his parents by the hands and do his own walking. Like all kids, sometimes he would try to break away and run off in a different direction.

Doug, who figured his son was just tired from all the excitement, hoisted

Jarrett into his arms and carried him to the car, strapped him in the back seat and drove home. Jarrett didn't say another word that night about feeling pain.

In Heaven, every day must be like a late September day in the Bluegrass State. Many of those days are just right—not too hot, not too cold. The rustling leaves, the light breezes, and the vibrant colors of the sky and trees in the early stages of change all combine for a few days to make life picture-perfect.

The day following the football game was like that. Doug spent the afternoon playing T-ball with Jarrett and Chelsea, the little girl who lived next door. They ran around in the backyard, wrestled, and played tag for a couple hours. Then, all of a sudden, Jarrett once again told his dad that his leg hurt.

"He wasn't crying," Doug said. "He just mentioned it was bothering him."

His parents decided Jarrett should take it easy the rest of the weekend. They weren't too alarmed but agreed if the boy's leg still nagged him on Monday, they would have their pediatrician check it out.

The next morning, the Mynears wanted to take Jarrett to see his grandmother, who lived seventy miles away in Louisville. Granny Jeanne, as Jarrett called her, woke early to spend the morning standing over the stove, preparing one of those Sunday meals grandmas do best. It would be a menu of comfort foods prepared in a kitchen perfumed with hot rolls and warm cookies. Granny couldn't wait to see her pride and joy. And she was eager to see how her daughter was "filling out." Jennifer had recently given her mother the good news that a second grandchild was on the way.

Jennifer bounced into Jarrett's room to get him ready for the trip. She pulled the covers off the little rascal and lifted him from the bed. As soon as she touched his feet to the floor, Jarrett let out a scream. Chills shot through Jennifer. It was if someone had jumped out at her in a dark alley. Goosebumps broke out on her arms.

She could tell by the look on Jarrett's face something was terribly wrong. His smile had turned into a scowl. She sat him back on the bed, and for just the third time in three days Jarrett said simply, "My leg hurts."

"I'll never forget it," Jennifer said. "I felt his right shin, and it was as hot as fire."

She got to a phone quickly and called their pediatrician. Because it was a Sunday, he wasn't in his office but he agreed to meet them there if they'd first go to Central Baptist Hospital for x-rays.

So the couple did what the doctor advised, and they all got together a couple of hours later. A quick exam of Jarrett had the doctor perplexed. It didn't appear any bones were broken or fractured, but he too felt the heat on the toddler's skin. His worst fear was that there was a bone infection. A little dark spot could be seen on the transparency.

"We were freaking out," Jennifer said. "Something in me, I guess a mother's intuition, told me it was serious. I was terribly frightened."

The pediatrician once again suggested a trip back to Central Baptist, this time for a blood test and a bone scan.

"I understood why he had wanted an x-ray," Doug said. "But a blood test? That didn't make sense to me."

The doctor went with them on the second trip.

"They had a little trouble finding a vein for the blood test, so they stuck Jarrett more than once," recalled Doug. "I was getting a little testy, wondering why they were doing this to a two-year-old—all that poking and prodding. But Jarrett never made a sound."

After the bone scan, the family pediatrician conferred with other doctors for what seemed to be hours.

To kill the time and search for comfort, Jennifer spent much of the afternoon making telephone calls from the hospital. Word that Jarrett was undergoing tests spread quickly among the family's many friends and relatives. Jennifer needed people to help keep her mind occupied and away from her worst fears. She still hadn't fully come to terms with her father's death fifteen months earlier. And she was two months into a complicated pregnancy. She wasn't sure she could deal with any more bad news.

Some of the people she called showed up at the hospital to offer moral support. All of them tried to be optimistic.

Jarrett's granny walked away from her Sunday dinner for four and drove to Lexington.

Finally, the medical professionals called the Mynears into a conference room, but they still had no clear idea as to what might be in Jarrett's leg. One thought it was indeed a bone infection. Another thought it was a tumor. They all agreed that a bone biopsy was needed first thing in the morning.

Monday again found the Mynears sitting for hours in a waiting room as Jarrett went under the knife.

"I remember Doug sitting there trying to read the doctors faces as they walked past the door," Jennifer said.

"He said, 'It doesn't look like they're going to give us bad news.' I wanted to believe him, but I couldn't.

"Finally, late in the afternoon, one of the doctors came out and said, 'There's good news and bad news. The good news is Jarrett made it through the surgery just fine. The bad news is there is a malignant tumor. We're ninety percent sure it's Ewing's sarcoma.'"

Jennifer felt the color flush from her face. Doug slumped down in his chair, feeling as if a heavy weight had just crashed down on his shoulders. The two had never felt so weak. In the coming months, they couldn't have been stronger.

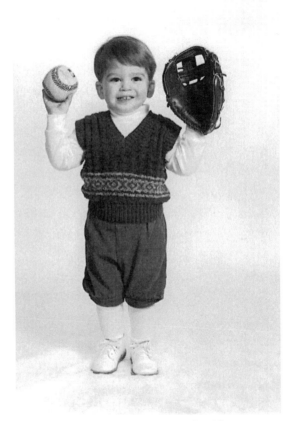

Jarrett at twenty months old

4

Diagnosis

Ewing's sarcoma is one of those mystery diseases. Medical experts don't know exactly what causes it. It's a bone cancer that's genetic but not hereditary.

The Mynears had no idea what the doctors were talking about when they mentioned the disease. There was just one pamphlet at the hospital entitled "Childhood Cancers," and it contained one sentence about Ewing's sarcoma. Later that night, the Mynears would go through a frantic and somewhat futile search for information at home, checking a medical dictionary and health-related software they had loaded on their computer.

Normal human cells contain twenty-three numbered pairs of chromosomes. In Ewing's sarcoma tumors, a piece of chromosome 11 has moved to chromosome 22, creating a new piece of DNA. Researchers know this so-called translocation often happens at a time of rapid growth. Children seem to be most vulnerable for tumor development in their teenage years, although the condition is extremely rare at any age.

Jarrett's doctors quickly discovered that he was one of the youngest people to ever develop the disease.

Ewing's sarcoma starts in the bone or soft tissue, usually in the pelvis or the thigh. Even a very small tumor can lead to a microscopic spread of the cancer. Therefore, the disease requires treatment to the whole body.

Dr. Jeffrey Parr, an orthopedic surgeon in Lexington, told the Mynears on that manic Monday that he wanted them to go to the Mayo Clinic to confirm his diagnosis. Parr had done his residency there and knew how to get Jarrett a quick appointment and whom he should see once he got there.

"We felt like we'd hit rock bottom," Jennifer said. "We were willing to do anything the doctors suggested, and the Mayo Clinic seemed like the best thing to do.

"But I just knew deep down inside that what we were hearing meant amputation at the very least."

By noon Wednesday, the family van was packed, and the Mynears were on the road for a fourteen-hour drive to Rochester, Minnesota. The most important cargo, besides Jarrett, of course, was a folder containing copies of the x-ray films and bone scans and slides of the tumor cells. During the long drive, Jarrett sat obliviously in the back seat, enjoying the passing scenery and clutching his favorite toy, a Raggedy Andy doll that was a gift from Granny Jeanne. Each time Jennifer looked back at him, she couldn't help but think they were taking their lamb to the lions.

They pulled into the parking lot of a Rochester motel at 2 A.M. As they stepped out of the car, the September air gave the threesome a cold welcome. In just five sleepless hours, they would have to be at the famous clinic. Doug and Jennifer felt as if their son were a defendant on trial, due in the courtroom first thing in the morning. The jury was set to consider the evidence. And even though little Jarrett had done nothing wrong, his parents knew the verdict could be devastating.

The Mayo Clinic operates with a team of two thousand physicians and sees more than a half million patients each year. Its excellent reputation for medical research is known around the world. But you aren't sent there for minor operations. If you're advised to go to Mayo, it's usually because your condition is so rare or so serious that your local doctors don't feel comfortable handling it alone.

"It's easy to see how people get intimidated there," Jennifer said. "That first morning we walked into a conference room to face an entire disciplinary team—a prosthetist, a physical therapist, oncology nurses, a child psychologist and social workers—all sitting there around a big conference table. We were overwhelmed.

"But as soon as the discussion started, we realized they were all there to help us. They made us feel as comfortable as humanly possible at such a stressful time. It was not impersonal at all, and we realized we needed to do whatever they advised."

For the next several hours, Jarrett was put through the wringer again. Even though the Mynears had the pathology slides and the x-rays from Lexington, the Mayo Clinic doctors wanted to repeat many of the tests. It started with a blood test, then a CAT scan and an MRI.

"It was the oddest thing," Jennifer said. 'From the beginning, Jarrett never cried. It was like an adventure for him. And that's not selective memory. The doctors were fascinated with his reaction."

Jarrett lay still as clinic aides strapped him to tables and poked him with needles. He just watched with curiosity as the modern medical machinery passed over his body, taking pictures of his insides. Just before Jarrett came into the CAT-scan room, another child had to be removed because he was kicking and screaming frantically. That boy's parents decided to schedule the procedure for another time when perhaps their young patient would be calmer and less frightened.

Jarrett's parents knew that despite the dreadfulness of the situation, they had a lot for which to be thankful. Their son's demeanor took the edge off a lot of difficult decisions.

"Jarrett could be hyper," Doug said. "But he was very workable. When he knew he had to lie still, he would. We never had to tell him twice."

Doctors said it was remarkable that at his age Jarrett didn't have to be put to sleep for the magnetic resonance imaging. Even though the MRI process is painless, children— and adults, for that matter—often feel claustrophobic as their body slides on a platform into the tube-shaped scanner. Any little wiggle could distort the final images.

The magnet can also emit loud banging and knocking noises that can cause people to flinch. But Jarrett stayed as still as a guard at Buckingham Palace.

Because of her pregnancy, Jennifer wasn't able to go into a lot of the examination rooms as Jarrett went through the battery of tests. So as Doug went from room to room with the doctors, she sat in the waiting room watching the second hand on a wall clock tick away the hours. She gazed at magazines but didn't really comprehend the articles. This wasn't like it had been in Lexington earlier in the week. Friends and relatives didn't surround her. She felt extremely lonely.

It was getting dark outside, and the doctors decided Jarrett had had enough for one day. They already had enough information to confirm the Kentucky diagnosis. This was indeed a case of Ewing's sarcoma. The doctors said they had one more procedure to do and then they'd let the family leave to go get some rest in their motel room.

Jennifer knew Doug had to be exhausted from being escorted all around the clinic for hours, so she told him she'd go with Jarrett for the final test. Admittedly, Doug was relieved to get a break, and he knew his wife would feel better about the situation if she spent some more time with Jarrett's doctors and nurses.

But neither of them was prepared for what happened next. They assumed it was going to be another blood test or some little end-of-the day evaluation.

"They told me to lay Jarrett down on his stomach," Jennifer said. "Then they said I'd have to hold his arms and lay my body down on his."

She was horrified to see them bring out a long hollow needle. They told her they needed to draw bone marrow from his pelvis. Jarrett was not sedated.

"Supposedly, it was easier on young patients not to take the time to knock them out," Jennifer said. "And they said someone that young can't always handle the heavy drugs it would take to ease the pain."

When the needle went into his pelvis, Jarrett broke his silence. The young man who had been a model patient all day let out a piercing scream. Then, a dam of emotions burst.

"He started to wail at the top of his lungs and squirm violently," Jennifer said. "The nurses were yelling at me to hold him still. I started to cry, and it was the worst feeling I've ever had. I knew my baby was in pain and I was allowing it to happen."

The door to the exam room was shut tight, but Doug could hear the commotion as he sat waiting on the other side. He jumped up and yelled frantically through the door, "What's going on in there?"

"Let me in . . . let me help . . . somebody tell me something!"

After the marrow was collected, Doug was allowed into the room. Mother, father, and son embraced in a group hug—three bodies shaking, three pairs of eyes wet.

It had to be done. They knew that. But they couldn't help feeling a little mad—mad at the doctors, mad at the world, maybe even mad at God.

As they packed up to leave for the evening, the Mynears picked up a Polaroid picture that had been taken of Jarrett that morning. He was wearing hospital scrubs and smiling the biggest smile you've ever seen. That was the image they wanted to carry home in their minds that night.

5

Sixty Days

Day Two at the Mayo Clinic had to be better than Day One. Most of the tests were over. Now it was just a matter of outlining the treatment.

The Mynears already knew Jarrett would have to go through chemotherapy. Before coming to Minnesota, they had spent several days in meetings, learning exactly how the process would work, how much it would cost, and about possible side effects. Those things were reiterated on the second day at Mayo and over the next several days, as doctors also discussed how Jarrett's diet would change and what medications he would receive.

The first item of the seventh day was to put the youngster into surgery so a catheter could be inserted under his skin. The quarter-sized disc, known as a port-o-cath, would supply an opening for a needle in the boy's abdomen, sparing his veins from repeated stabbings.

As she waited for Jarrett to come out of the recovery room, Jennifer began to think about all the gifts her son had received at the beginning of the week when he first went in for tests in Lexington. She knew more would be coming. Everyone who knew Jarrett loved him, and they wanted to make him feel better. Of course, toys and trinkets, cards and candy would do that.

"I knew it would be hard to maintain some kind of discipline," Jennifer said. "I didn't want to deny him anything, but I also didn't want him to become a spoiled brat. And I didn't want him to use his condition to get his way."

Jennifer and Doug had a meeting with a child psychologist at the clinic that day, and Jennifer expressed her concern that Jarrett might feel sorry for himself and become a source of pity. She worried that too much sympathy might make him manipulative or cause him to give up fending for himself.

The psychologist asked to spend some time with Jarrett and was granted a one-on-one appointment that afternoon.

After spending about a half-hour with Jarrett, the counselor came out and had a simple but profound statement for his parents: "He's going to be the one to get *you* through this. I can tell from his determination and intelligence that he's going to be the strong one. You have nothing to worry about."

Relief washed over the Mynears like a spring rain.

It's hard to describe a roller coaster unless you've been on one. You know it goes up and down, fast and slow, but until you've felt your stomach in your throat and the breath knocked out of you, you really have no idea what the ride is like.

The Mynears were on an emotional roller coaster, and each time they thought things were looking up, the track twisted, plunging them again into a tunnel or turning their outlook upside down.

When they went to their motel room after a second day at the clinic, they found a blinking red light on the telephone, meaning they had a message. They dialed a special code to hear what was recorded.

"Doug, Jennifer," said the voice from a friend back home. "I know you've got a lot on your mind and I hate to tell you this, but you need to know. The front door of your house is wide open, and there's a knife in the deadbolt. Someone broke in last night."

The roller coaster knocked the wind out of them again.

The frustration and helplessness the Mynears felt by their son's illness was now compounded with a feeling of violation. Were they going to have to endure the trials of Job? It's been said God never gives you more than you can handle, but the Mynears were beginning to wonder.

They called the friend back home, who described the scene. The intruder had tried to chop the deadbolt out of the front door. When that didn't work, he or she had apparently kicked the door down. Inside their home, every drawer to every desk, cabinet, and dresser had been ransacked.

After a few minutes of collecting their wits about them, the couple began placing calls to family members, spending much of the evening making arrangements for their home to be secured. Of course, they told each other it wouldn't matter if all their possessions were gone. What really mattered was in that hotel room—mother, father, son, and baby-to-be.

Even years later, they weren't able to determine if anything was actually stolen. Cameras, television sets and jewelry were left untouched. No one was ever arrested. There was no clue as to why the burglar tore through their belongings. But the Mynears had to stay in Minnesota twelve more days, and all that time they were nervous about what they'd find when they returned home.

On the third day at Mayo, the feared announcement came. Option A was also Option B, C, and D. The doctors said, with finality, that the only way to get rid of Jarrett's cancer was to administer chemotherapy and take off his right leg from the knee down. Other options open to older patients weren't available for Jarrett. Radiation of the tumor site would've killed the growth plates in his leg, freezing it permanently to the size of a two-year-old. And limb-sparing replacement surgery wasn't an alternative for someone who'd barely begun to grow.

Jennifer's intuition was right, but it was still difficult to hear that actual surgery was imminent. Doctors arranged for Jarrett to come back in two months for an amputation.

During the next week at the clinic, bone experts fitted Jarrett with a leg brace that went from the heel of his right foot all the way to the top of his hip. They said the tumor in his fibula had grown, making his leg extremely fragile. The hard plastic brace immobilized the leg so Jarrett couldn't bend his knee or put his full weight down on that foot. The boy had to learn to walk by swinging the brace in a large arc, then taking a normal step with his left leg. At first, straight paths were nearly impossible, but he took the new stride in stride, again showing pride in the way he could tackle a challenge.

The day before leaving the hospital, Jarrett had his first chemotherapy treatment. He sat for hours as poison dripped into his little veins, killing cancerous cells and growth cells, too.

That liquid trickling down the intravenous tube was the real burglar in the Mynears' lives. It was robbing their son of a normal childhood, taking away so much more than any two-bit vandal could ever steal from their house. But the droplets also carried hope, an expectation that the cancer was being stopped in its tracks.

Jennifer and Doug watched as Jarrett took it all in, asking questions about the "stuff" the nurses kept pouring in the bottles connected to the tube that went into his body.

"What's that?"

"How much do I need?"

"Will it make me pee?"

He greeted everyone who came in and out of the room and smiled and waved to each one who left. The child psychologist was right. This kid wasn't about to be robbed of his spirit.

Jarrett vomited in the hospital room that night and again after breakfast the next morning. But it wasn't a prolonged reaction. Experts say children generally tolerate chemotherapy better than adults do. Most times in the months after that, the boy showed no signs of sickness after a treatment.

Following the failed attempt to give Jarrett some food for the road, the Mynears packed up the van and headed home to Kentucky. They'd been away two weeks that seemed like two months. They were road warriors returning from battle, but the war was just beginning.

Mommy and Daddy had sixty days to prepare their son for the loss of his leg and what would become routine hospital stays. They would also have to prepare themselves.

6

Amputation

October brought some nice days to Central Kentucky, sunny afternoons when father and son could stroll outside. As Jarrett kicked at the leaves on the ground, Doug couldn't help but think this would be the last autumn for that. Even though his boy was hindered by a brace, he could still move at a pretty quick pace, sending neatly piled leaves into fluttering disarray. It was fun to watch.

When November snow covered the ground, the boy's footprints in the yard made a trail of tears for his parents. It wasn't as if Jarrett would never walk again. His parents knew he would, but it wouldn't be his real foot trampling the blankets of white.

Jarrett lost all of his hair before Thanksgiving, but that didn't seem to bother him. He thought he looked like the Kung Fu masters he saw on TV.

Doug and Jennifer talked to their son about the pending amputation and tried to be as upbeat as they could. They told him how it would take the hurt away and get all the cancer out of his body, that he would be healthy again, and that it wouldn't stop him from doing anything he wanted to do in life. They told him he would be *unique* and that other kids would be amazed by his artificial leg. And most importantly, they kept a notebook for Jarrett, writing down any questions he wanted to ask the doctors.

They were the kind of questions you would expect a kid to ask:

1. How are they going to cut off my leg?
2. What kind of tools will they use?
3. What will they do with my leg?

The third question made Doug and Jennifer laugh out loud. They wanted to know about things such as infection and painkillers. Their son wanted to make sure his leg wasn't going to be turned into a lamp.

Jarrett's treatment protocol called for a chemotherapy session every three weeks. Mayo Clinic arranged for those to take place at the University of Kentucky Hospital. It was a routine that would continue for a year. Doctors said that's how long it would take to make sure the boy's body was cancer-free.

Just after Thanksgiving, the Mynears headed for Rochester, Minnesota, again, this time taking a free flight offered by Continental Airlines.

A shuttle picked them up at the airport and took them to a nicer hotel than the one they had stayed in before, much closer to the clinic. All of the arrangements were better this time. Jarrett was now a known client of the highly-respected Mayo Clinic, and provisions had been made to make his second visit as comfortable as possible.

But the welcome still seemed unfriendly, not because of the people but because of the circumstances. Doug remembered how dreary the sky seemed.

"There was a foot of snow on the ground, and the wind chill was forty below," he said.

"We would've rather been anywhere else. It was a tough thing knowing our son was coming here to be changed forever."

The next day they met Dr. Michael Rock, the orthopedic surgeon who would perform the amputation. He came equipped with impressive credentials, but Doug wasn't sure he liked him.

"He didn't make a great first impression," Doug said. "He seemed so businesslike and stern. We weren't sure he could relate to plain folks from Kentucky."

Dr. Rock was indeed all business when he first consulted with the threesome. "Cut and dry" is how Jennifer would describe the doctor's demeanor.

"He was talking directly to Doug and me. There was no interaction with Jarrett at all. In the middle of the appointment, Jarrett decided he'd had enough.

"He was very articulate. We wanted him to show good manners, but we understood when he spoke up and said, 'Hey, I'm the one having my leg cut off. You need to talk to me!'"

The outburst caught Dr. Rock by surprise. He hadn't meant to slight the patient. He just wasn't used to children under the age of three paying such close attention to discussions of medical procedures.

"Dr. Rock turned around and looked straight at Jarrett," Jennifer said. "I thought things were about to get tense. I figured he'd say, 'Son, mind your own business. I'm talking to your parents.'

"Instead, he apologized and told Jarrett he had made a good point. Then he went through Jarrett's list of questions, answering each one in a way a child could understand. From that day on, they were the best of buddies. Jarrett had input in all the meetings after that."

Doug's concerns also disappeared immediately. "Our initial view of Dr. Rock was wrong," he said. "He was great through the whole thing."

Doug and Jennifer learned that just prior to Jarrett's visit to Mayo for the surgery, he may have been exposed to chickenpox. So this stint in the hospital was going to be lonelier. Even though he showed no signs of the childhood virus, he would have to stay in isolation, away from other kids and out of the playroom. He couldn't even be taken into the hallways.

But toys came to the room, wrapped in plastic. Jarrett passed the hours in a fantasy world of his own, playing with action figures and model cars, building towers with blocks and filling the pages of coloring books. When the toys went back to the playroom, they were sterilized.

"When the day of surgery came, we thought we were ready for it," Jennifer said. "But . . .," she paused, her voice breaking up, ". . . there's no way to describe what goes through your mind when you're going into the operating ward."

"That was the first time it really, I mean *really,* sunk in for me," Doug said. "You keep thinking things will change."

Jarrett was given a hospital gown and slippers. Aides wheeled him away on a gurney, as his parents watched from their seats in a waiting area, not taking their eyes off the procession until it rounded a corner out of their view.

A few minutes later, an aide came back, carrying one slipper; the one Jarrett wouldn't need for a right foot. She handed it to Jennifer, who immediately broke down in tears. She leaned her head over on Doug's shoulder, and then he lost it, too.

Imagine the scene as a bystander. Here was a couple distraught, caught up in a deeply personal, emotional moment. You have no idea what the pregnant woman and her husband are going through, but you feel your eyes tearing up, too. You wish you could say something to make it better, but nothing comes to mind. You hurt for them. The air is heavy with sadness. The man's shirt is wet from his wife's sobs.

"It was the only insensitive thing we experienced there," Jennifer said. "I wish they had kept that slipper."

After a grueling three-hour wait, the parents were allowed to see their son. He was asleep, covered with a blanket. Again, like so many times before, Jennifer and Doug told themselves they could handle what they were about to see.

"But when they pulled the blanket down and the leg was missing, it was another emotional round for me," Jennifer said.

She wondered just how much water could be left in her tear ducts.

Doug spent the night at the hospital, holding Jarrett's hand and listening to his steady breathing. The boy was "conked out," heavily medicated with morphine for pain relief. Jennifer tried to get some sleep at the hotel. Easier said than done.

The next night, it was Jennifer's turn to stay at the hospital. The hours were long and boring as she lay on a cot staring at the ceiling, tracing the plastered patterns with her eyes. She munched on candy as her mind swirled with thoughts about what lay ahead for her son.

"I want some of those Junior Mints."

A squeaky whisper broke the silence.

Jennifer looked over at the bed and Jarrett was looking back, wide awake and smiling. His first concern was his hungry stomach, not his missing leg.

The operation was a through-the-knee disarticulation. The surgeons didn't separate bone, just muscle and ligaments. That way, when the lower leg was removed, no jagged bone was left.

Jarrett had been fitted with a cast that went over the part of his leg that remained. It had a metal joint on the end, a place to affix a prosthesis.

After he downed his Junior Mints and enjoyed some kisses and cuddling from his mother, Jarrett suddenly seemed to become aware for the first time that his body wasn't the same as it had been two days earlier.

"He was upset when he kicked the covers down," Jennifer said. "He thought his leg was folded up in the cast. I had to remind him that his leg was gone and that he'd see that when the cast was removed."

The experts didn't make a permanent prosthesis at first because of the swelling. The artificial leg was crude, to say the least, fashioned out of plastic PVC pipe, the kind you use to run water lines into your house.

On the third day after the surgery, the nurses brought Jarrett a tiny walker and he took his first steps on the plastic leg. He was totally off his pain medication then and eager to move around his room. Again, he saw it as a challenge. His parents gave him applause and encouragement with each step, and Jarrett ate it up. It was like a child showing off when he first learns to ride a bike or stand on his head.

"We told him how proud we were," Jennifer said. "And we meant it."

Again, they had evidence all around them to illustrate how well Jarrett was adapting to the circumstances. A teenage girl at the clinic had gone in for the same surgery at the same time as Jarrett. She too had lost a leg to Ewing's sarcoma. She was still bedridden and taking heavy doses of morphine when Jarrett was shuffling around his room, demonstrating his new way of walking to anyone who would watch.

Because of the chickenpox scare, Jarrett couldn't take long strolls during the day. He still had to stay isolated in his room. But each night for the next week, his dad carried him up a back stairway to the psychiatric ward. An empty hallway there gave the young man all the room he needed to practice stepping out.

Physical therapists came in during the day, giving Jarrett an exercise regimen. The temporary artificial leg didn't bend, so they knew it would take time for the boy to really get the feel of it and find his balance.

"They said he'd need the walker for three months," Jennifer said. "But three weeks later, he put that walker in a corner and pretty much never used it again."

Two days before Christmas, Jarrett got to leave the Mayo Clinic. He had to be home in time for Santa Claus.

The hospital staff, still concerned that Jarrett may carry the chickenpox virus, cleared the hallways so the boy could be taken to the checkout desk. As his wheelchair turned a corner, Jarrett spotted a familiar face.

He yelled, at the top of his lungs, "There's the man who cut my leg off!"

Nurses popped their heads out of doorways, obviously alarmed.

Then Jarrett put on the biggest smile he could muster and waved his hand wildly.

"Hey, Dr. Rock. Good to see you!"

The hallway echoed with laughter.

7
Adjustment

Christmas at Granny's house in Louisville was "Jarrett's Day." There's no doubt about it. He was the center of attention.

Jennifer's twin brothers Chris and Mike, whom she described as "trying to be tough and macho," softened quite a bit when they saw Jarrett. They showered their nephew with gifts and tried their best to act as if nothing had changed. They wrestled with the boy, gave him piggyback rides, and sat with him to watch the holiday football games on television, explaining the plays to him and telling him when they thought the referees had made a bad call.

Everyone encouraged Jarrett to show off how well he could get around with his prosthesis. And he was happy to oblige. The living room was an obstacle course, with a large Christmas tree and stacks of gifts to maneuver around, but Jarrett strutted the length of the room again and again, and basked in the applause and praise each time.

Granny had made more cookies than usual, and Jarrett was allowed to have as many as he wanted. And throughout the day, he talked about his visit the night before from Saint Nick.

Jarrett hadn't been able to go to the mall to see Santa that year, and that concerned him greatly. His mother assured him that his wish list made it to the North Pole anyway, but in true fashion, Jarrett would've liked to have spoken to the man directly.

On Christmas Eve, as the family was making last-minute preparations for the trip to Granny's house, there was a knock at the door of their Lexington home. They heard the sound of jingling bells coming from the porch. Jarrett's parents told him to go see who was there.

When he opened it, he let out a cry of delight. Santa Claus stood there with gifts in his arms.

"I knew you couldn't come see me this year, so I came to see you," Santa said. "I know you've been a very good boy."

Santa sat in a big chair in the living room, and Jarrett climbed onto his lap.

"Thank you for coming," Jarrett said. "I knew you wouldn't forget me."

Doug's best friend, David Crowell, had arranged for a co-worker to don the red suit, and the colleague looked great in the fake beard and shiny boots. His appearance seemed so real that even the adults half expected to see reindeer on the lawn.

Everyone watched intently as Jarrett pulled the wrapping and bows off each gift. The comfort and joy the family felt reminded them more than ever that Christmas was a time of miracles.

The prayer before the big turkey dinner the next day touched each person around the table. It was a "thank you" to God for a child born more than two thousand years ago and for the child in the room.

Continuing his chemotherapy treatments in the months that followed, Jarrett had a visit to the UK Children's Hospital every third weekend. Doug and Jennifer would switch off each trip, which required going in on Friday and staying overnight.

Jarrett was also at the clinic in between chemo treatments for physical therapy, blood counts, and transfusions. Doug's father, known to Jarrett as "Paw," became a well-known figure around the pediatric ward. He would go with Jennifer every time, helping carry Jarrett from the car and into the treatment rooms. The boy was getting heavy, and Jennifer had another child on the way.

The stress of the previous months really began to wear on Jennifer that spring. Her pregnancy caused great discomfort, and she didn't sleep well. The thought of another impromptu rush to the hospital was extremely unsettling. So, her doctor scheduled a C-section for March 4, 1992, taking the guesswork out of when and where the birth would take place. Any structure in life was good at this point.

So that day Jarrett became a big brother. His sister Claire entered the family. But he wasn't there to greet her when she came home for the first time. He was back at the clinic with his dad. It was a chemo weekend.

At that point, Doug had to give Jarrett shots for ten nights in a row after each chemo treatment. They were Granulocyte Colony Stimulating Factor (G-CSF) shots, which contained a blood stimulant for building up the immune system. They cost $150 each, but they kept Jarrett from getting infections. The shots made his white cell count soar so he'd be able to take the next round of chemo. His parents and the insurance company would work out payment later. They couldn't allow themselves to think about the mounting bills right then.

Jarrett came to dread the nightly shots to the upper thigh, and Doug had to bribe him to sit still.

"He had been poked and prodded so much, and he just wasn't convinced that more shots would make a difference," Doug said. "I'd give him a quarter after each shot, and he would accept that as proper payment."

One month after Claire's birth, Jarrett was due back at the Mayo Clinic for restaging. That meant another round of the tests they had all become so familiar with—x-rays, an MRI, a CAT scan, and blood counts. Jennifer stayed behind with the baby while Doug, Jarrett, and Paw drove to Minnesota.

It was a happy visit. All the tests came back with good results.

"It really looked like we had killed the cancer," Doug said. "We were supposed to continue with the chemotherapy until September, just in case, but it appeared everything would be a breeze after that."

The next six months did indeed seem easy compared to what they'd been through. Jarrett turned three. The chemo visits became routine. And the young man became somewhat of a star patient around the hospital.

The nurses would come running to make over him each time he checked in. They joked with him, and one kept a squirt gun handy, always ready to give Jarrett a playful spray when he wasn't looking.

"They kept him keyed up while he was there," Doug said. "They were used to seeing so many sad children that Jarrett was a joy for them to work with."

"One resident even brought her husband in to meet Jarrett," Doug added. "She had been trying to convince him they should have children and she wanted him to see how much fun it was to be around Jarrett."

Jarrett wouldn't eat breakfast at the hospital. He saved his appetite. Father and son made it a ritual to go for pizza each Saturday afternoon after checkout. While eating the pepperoni and cheese treat, they'd count down how many more times they'd do the same thing.

"We really could see the light at the end of the tunnel," Doug said.

One day shortly after Claire's birth, Jennifer drove down Lexington's Southland Drive, one of the city's older business districts. She had driven the route hundreds of times but never noticed the sign before.

"ARTIFICIAL LIMBS" just jumped out at her in big block letters.

Jennifer and Doug were at a point where they had to make a decision about Jarrett's prosthesis. The crude PVC pipe had outlived its usefulness. The swelling above the right knee was down, and Jarrett had healed from the amputation.

"I just pulled my car in there to talk with them," Jennifer said. "It was on a whim, but I had a lot of questions."

His parents could have worked through a hospital to get Jarrett a new leg, but the folks at Hi-Tech Artificial Limbs just seemed to be the contact they needed.

"They were a godsend," Jennifer said. "I feel I was guided there."

The company offered a private place where she could take Jarrett, avoiding long hours in hospital rooms and multiple consultations with yet another team of doctors.

When Jennifer took Jarrett to Hi-Tech, the experts there made points by talking directly to Jarrett, asking him what he would like his new leg to be able to do.

"I want my leg to bend," Jarrett said. "I want to be able to sit at a table."

With his temporary leg, Jarrett had to sit on a booster seat or have his leg extended straight out on another chair. It really did limit his ability to eat with other people, to run and climb like any other three-year-old, or work in his activity books while seated.

Jarrett hit it off immediately with Maurice Adkins, Hi-Tech's president, maybe because the two had so much in common. Maurice had a prosthesis, too, attached at the same point on his right leg were Jarrett's limb would be connected.

"And we were both bald, and we both liked old cars," said Maurice, whose office was lined with pictures of classic coupes he had refurbished.

Over the years, Maurice, a man who could've been Jarrett's grandfather, became one of his best friends. He was a confidant and a spiritual advisor.

Maurice's right leg had been shattered in 1973 when he was working on the railroad near his mountain home in Pike County in the far southeastern tip of Kentucky. Two trains collided, spilling a load of lumber onto Maurice. A board pierced completely through his shin as he lay trapped underneath the crushing weight.

He had a religious conversion under that pile of boards, praying like he had never prayed before, and he was an outspoken Christian from that moment on, willing to talk about his faith to anyone who would listen.

He and Jarrett had many deep discussions over the years, about life and death, business and the Bible, faith and friendship.

Not a week went by that Maurice didn't get together with his little buddy. For more than ten years, they had a weekly dinner date, usually for pizza or tacos. If Jarrett was in the hospital, then they would have their meals together there. The only time the routine was thrown off was when Jarrett was out of state for treatment. Even then, Maurice made weekly phone calls.

That's why Jennifer called her discovery of that little office on Southland Drive a "godsend."

A leg that fit Jarrett's specifications was ordered and made in less than a month.

"When they put it on him for the first time and he sat down in a chair and it bent, he almost cried," his mother said. "He was so excited. He just kept talking about how now he could sit down like the rest of the kids."

Almost immediately, he got into running and climbing, making his parents happy and nervous at the same time.

"We thought he was active before," Jennifer said. "Now, we were about to find out what active really meant."

The chemo treatments ended in September, and the family asked Jarrett how he would like to celebrate. Not surprisingly, he wanted to meet Chip and Dale, the polite chipmunks who were central characters in many of his books and videotapes. So Jennifer and Doug dipped into a rainy day fund and cut a few corners on household expenses to make Jarrett's dream vacation possible.

It seemed as if he had stored up three-and-a-half years' worth of energy when they went to Walt Disney World, and it all came pouring out as he strolled through the Magic Kingdom. He wanted to ride every ride, see every show, and shake hands with every costumed character.

It was a tiring trip for Doug, Jennifer, Granny Jeanne and Jarrett, but a good kind of tired. As they rode the monorail out of the park late that night, Jarrett's head rested on his mother's arm. He fell asleep wearing plastic mouse ears and the smile of a Cheshire cat.

The next January, Jarrett went to preschool at a local church.

"We thought it was time to get him back into a normal routine," Jennifer said. "He had been basically isolated from his peers for more than a year."

He couldn't start in August like the other children because his chemo treatments didn't end until September. His parents didn't want him to start back to school in the middle of the term, and they elected to wait until January. Just before Christmas, Jennifer and Doug took him to check out the school, and once again his arrival at a new place stood out.

"He walked around like he owned the place," his mother said.

"He went right up to the teachers and said, 'My name is Jarrett Mynear and I'm going to be in your class.'"

"I've had cancer, but I'm better now," he added matter-of-factly.

The teachers laughed at his outgoing personality. Typically, he had dozens of questions. He wanted to know where he would sit, where he would hang his coat and keep his supplies and what kind of snacks they served. He was clearly excited.

On the first day of the January session, Jennifer arranged with the teachers to come in with Jarrett and have a talk with the other preschoolers.

They explained why Jarrett didn't have much hair (it was just beginning to grow back) and why there would be days he would not be able to come to school. He showed them how his leg could come off and how he could turn it around for comic effect. He was forty-four months old, with a better knack for public speaking than many forty-four-year-olds.

"He was never ashamed of it or self-conscious," Jennifer said. "I sat there for moral support, but Jarrett really presented the lesson. He answered any questions the kids had. I wasn't worried any more about his social skills after that."

Jarrett truly loved going to preschool and pouted on the days when he couldn't go. His parents had to pull him out for weeks at a time whenever there was an outbreak of chickenpox. He still wasn't healthy enough to be immunized.

"We had to explain to him why it was O.K. for the other kids to break out in a rash but not for him," Jennifer said. "Chickenpox could've killed him."

But, except for that fear that he'd contract a childhood virus, life seemed back on track.

Jennifer went back to work part-time as a teacher at Paul Laurence Dunbar High School. It was good for her to get her mind back on her career.

Jarrett turned four, finished the spring session of preschool, and headed back to the Mayo Clinic for his twenty-one-month checkup.

"The doctors there were excited to see him. They went through all the tests and scans and were beaming when they gave us the results," Jennifer said.

"The word they used was 'awesome,'" she said. "They said there's a better than ninety percent chance Jarrett had been cured. Basically, they told us to go back to Kentucky and have a nice life."

One of the doctors came to the examining room to ask Jarrett for a favor. He said there was a couple in the hallway whose daughter was facing an amputation, and they had a lot of concerns about how it would affect her mobility. The doctor wanted Jarrett to demonstrate how well he could run with a prosthetic leg.

Jarrett said he'd be glad to, and he instantly kicked into a "show off" mode. He ran up and down the hall, not once but three times, making sharp turns on his heels when he changed direction and picking up speed each time, giggling all the way.

Doug and Jennifer saw relief on the faces of the mother and father who were about to send their child under the knife. Two strangers suddenly realized they could handle the ordeal they were about to confront. At that moment, their son was a counselor, providing encouragement to a man and woman desperately in need of cheer. It was a role he would take on many times in the years to come.

Jarrett spent the summer doing what four-year-olds do—drawing pictures, watching television, playing baseball with his dad, and pulling pranks on his babysitters.

One Saturday, just as the family was getting ready to drive to Granny Jeanne's house in Louisville, the phone rang.

Jennifer's mother was on the line, asking her to have Doug bring rubber gloves to her house.

"Why in the world would he need to bring rubber gloves?" Jennifer asked.

"Well, there's a little mess to clean up," her mother said.

When they got to the house, they discovered a dead tree frog on Granny Jeanne's bedroom floor. Her house was surrounded by trees that towered over the roof, and apparently a frog had fallen down the chimney in the night.

When Jeanne awoke that morning, she saw the frog staring at her from atop a stack of books on her nightstand. She shrieked and swiped at the frog, knocking it and the books to the floor. A book fell on the little amphibian, flattening it on the carpet.

"Jarrett could just imagine his grandmother's rash reaction when she saw the frog, and he thought it was funny," Jennifer said. "He teased her, saying, 'Granny is a frog killer.' It became something he joked about with her from that day forward."

Any time Jarrett saw a plastic or ceramic tree frog in a toy store or gift shop, he wanted to buy it for his granny. And she returned the favor, buying him fake frogs. When one of the two presented a gift bag to the other, the recipient knew before opening the bag there was likely a frog inside. It was a human connection using toys—a concept that would someday be Jarrett's claim to fame.

Jarrett completed another session of preschool the following fall and spring. For a full year, the roller coaster stayed parked at the station. Medically, his life was uneventful. The checkups that came every three months continued to bring good news. Cancer appeared to be something he had whipped.

As his kindergarten season approached, his family couldn't have known the coaster was about to plunge again.

8

The Cancer Returns

By all appearances, the Mynears had been given a fresh start. They had decided their house in Lexington was too small for their growing family and found a place they loved on an acre just two miles to the south in Jessamine County. It was near woods and fields—good places for kids to explore.

Jarrett went to kindergarten in a new place, but he didn't act like a stranger. Once again, he started the year by telling his new classmates at Rosenwald-Dunbar Elementary School about his cancer and his artificial leg. But by then, he was talking as a cancer survivor, telling them it was all gone.

"There's nothing to worry about," he told the other four- and five-year olds. "You can't catch it. It's not like the mumps or chickenpox. And even if that were possible, you wouldn't catch it from me. I don't have it anymore."

But, unknowingly, Jarrett told a lie.

One evening, about a month into the term, Doug helped Jarrett get ready for bed. As he shampooed Jarrett's hair, which was now thick and dark, he noticed a tender spot on the crown of his head.

"Ouch!" Jarrett winced, as his dad touched it again.

"He was a very active kid, so we thought he had bumped it on the playground or on something at school," Doug said. "But Jarrett said he couldn't remember hitting anything with his head."

His parents checked the spot for about five days, and it didn't get any better. Experience told them they'd better see a doctor.

A trip to the UK Hospital revealed the last thing anyone wanted to hear. There was a tumor under that soft spot on Jarrett's skull.

Once again, they packed the family van and headed to the Mayo Clinic, this time with toddler Claire in tow and Granny Jeanne along to baby-sit.

"They pulled all the scans from June, and it was there, "Jennifer said in disbelief. "They had missed it!"

A dark spot showed up on the slides of Jarrett's skull, and somehow the best doctors in the world at one of the best clinics in the world had overlooked it. The scans had been taken from the front and back of the skull but not from the top. It's important to remember that Jarrett was one of the youngest patients ever diagnosed with Ewing's sarcoma, so there wasn't any history on how to best test for the spread of the disease in someone his age.

Typically, Ewing's goes from the arms and legs into the lungs. Over the years, doctors have learned they better check everywhere. Now, they always do a scan of the top of the head.

"We couldn't believe it wasn't caught," Jennifer said.

She admits that she was instantly angry. How could they be going through this again? If they had noticed this four months ago, could it have been nipped in the bud?

"But after you go through being mad and settle down, you realize everyone's human," Jennifer said. "Nobody's perfect. These things happen. The past can't be changed. You just have to concentrate on what's next."

The doctors devised another treatment plan.

"The specialist on the case made the statement that he wanted to go at it full force and get rid of this thing once and for all," Jennifer said.

"Full force" meant a three-month regimen of super intensive chemotherapy back at UK. Jarrett was in the hospital five days at a time for these strong treatments, which again came every three weeks.

Jennifer took a leave of absence from her half-day teaching job so she could be at the hospital during those five-day stretches. Claire had to be shuttled to a babysitter every day while Doug worked because the Mynears didn't want another child to have to spend countless hours around doctors, nurses, and sick people.

Their good friend Julie Hoagland became like Claire's big sister. She was the ever-dependable babysitter, always available and never concerned about ˙long the family would be away.

ʔt me from completely losing my mind," Jennifer said. "It was hard for me to leave Claire every day, but I knew she was with someone who genuinely loved her and treated her like her own child. She was much more than just a babysitter. She was part of the family."

Doug would relieve Jennifer at the end of his workday, so the couple spent very little time together.

"We would meet for dinner in Jarrett's room, and then one would go home with Claire and the other would stay at the hospital with Jarrett," Doug said. "It was a lonely time for all of us."

After the three months of chemo ended, doctors still had no assurance they were beating the cancer. When pressed for a prognosis, the doctors said Jarrett had about a five-percent chance of living with conventional treatments. So, another big decision fell into the Mynears' laps.

"They told us the best chance for getting rid of the cancer forever was to do a stem cell transplant," Jennifer said. "And the best place for that would be the Fred Hutchinson Cancer Research Center in Seattle.

"That would mean uprooting and moving clear across the country for several months," she said. "But that's just an automatic. You do what you need to do."

Stem cell transplant. Another new term. They didn't like the sound of it.

Jennifer said, "We read and read until we were cross-eyed, but that still doesn't prepare you for what it really means."

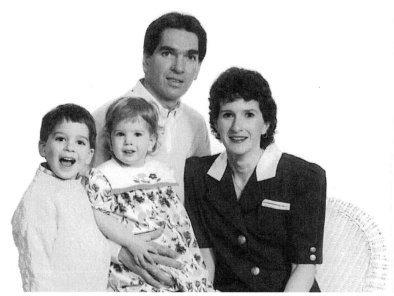

Mynear family portrait: Jarrett, Claire, Doug and Jennifer

9

Sickness in Seattle

Stem cells are baby blood cells that haven't decided what they will be when they grow up. They could become red cells (which carry oxygen around the body), white cells (which protect against infection), or platelets (which prevent bleeding).

In Jarrett's case, the doctors wanted an autologous transplant. That meant the stem cells would come from his own bloodstream. Getting them from him was less risky procedure than using donated cells, which could carry disease or trigger a negative reaction.

The cells would be taken from a special catheter in Jarrett's chest, stored while he underwent a strong chemo session to kill his bone marrow and then returned to his body. If all worked as planned, the returned baby cells would travel through the bloodstream and find their way to the bone marrow, where they would start to grow and develop into mature blood cells. He would be injected with growth factors to encourage the stem cells to migrate from the marrow into the bloodstream.

All of the literature told the Mynears this could be highly beneficial. But they also read that the process had side effects in people who are in generally poor health, and each year about one in four patients die from the procedure.

They had faced a lot of tough decisions, but none of them had seemed to be matters of life and death. They were having brainstorms, but not the kind that reflect sudden great ideas. These were the kind of storms that cloud your thinking, give you headaches, and keep you awake at night. It was as if a flood of thoughts was rushing around in their turbulent heads, none of them secure enough to grasp.

The doctors had made a mistake months earlier when they missed the tumor on a brain scan. Now they recommended a risky transplant. Did they really know or were they guessing? Was their son being used as a guinea pig?

The doctors' voices grew stronger as they echoed in Doug and Jennifer's minds. *"Jarrett is young and active." "He can fight off any side effects." "The fatalities happen to older people." "Trust us. Trust us. Trust us."*

"We really came to the conclusion that we had no choice but to trust them," Jennifer said.

"God gave us a child to take care of, and now we had to turn his well-being over to total strangers. That's where helplessness came in."

Jennifer and Doug found out what it means to be "talked out." They discussed every scenario with each other until they couldn't think of anything else to say. They prayed more than they had ever prayed. And, despite continued trepidation, the answer seemed to be clear. They would go to Seattle and once again meet more doctors they had never seen before at another world-renowned institution.

The day after Thanksgiving, the family of four boarded a plane bound for the West Coast but with no guarantee the Fred Hutchinson Center would even take Jarrett as a patient.

Doug brought along a laptop computer. He had arranged to transfer a lot of his work with him. It was truly amazing how understanding his employer was and how willing his bosses at Booker Associates were to work around his complicated lifestyle.

On the following Monday, the Mynears showed up at the cancer center— a pristine building in a beautiful city. It was a change in longitude and latitude, but everything else was deja vu.

Inside, it could have been Any Hospital U.S.A. The machinery looked the same, the needles were just as sharp and the smells and noises told you this was a place for sick people. Jarrett went through the familiar battery of tests— being dabbed with syringes, scanned with magnets and photographed with bursts of radiation.

By the end of the week, the specialists there said they would admit Jarrett to the clinic and proceed with the stem cell harvest. Again, the doctors tried to assure the Mynears that this was *the* way to go.

That evening, the Kentucky clan checked into a three-hundred-square foot efficiency apartment just a few blocks from the cancer center. It was way too crowded for four people, but the price was right and the location convenient. But, Doug and Jennifer knew it would mostly be a place to sleep. They would be at the hospital almost every waking hour.

They were used to these trips away from home being miserable. This time, Claire got the blahs. She had developed some type of breathing infection just before they left home. She sat around feeling dismal most of the time. Her parents felt helpless, wishing they could wave a magic wand and make their little girl bouncy and playful.

This initial trip to Seattle was expected to take five to seven days. Each day, Jarrett showed up to have his blood counts tested. The stem cells would be collected when everything was at the right level. He received daily shots to stimulate his white count, but a week passed and the count just wasn't high enough.

They stayed an extra week before doctors attempted the harvest.

On the appointed day, Jarrett stretched out on a bed and went to sleep under heavy anesthetics. A drip was stuck into a vein just under his collarbone. Blood traveled from his body and trickled into a centrifuge, which spun rapidly to separate the stem cells. The remaining blood returned to him through the drip in another vein. The process lasted nearly four hours, with the collected stem cells being immediately frozen. They would be saved until after Jarrett had gone through another round of high-dose chemotherapy.

But the process was only semi-successful. It didn't yield nearly enough cells. The family learned Jarrett would have to stay at the center a few more days, until his white count got high enough to try again.

After another week of low counts, the Mynears temporarily put the red light on the procedure.

"It was getting closer to Christmas, and we had two kids who were getting very fidgety," Jennifer said. "They were both very much into Christmas, and none of us could stand another day in that efficiency apartment.

"Friends had been sending us cards and miniature Christmas trees that were all decorated and that just made us all the more homesick."

They flew back to Kentucky in time to spend the holiday with the whole family—grandparents, aunts and uncles, nieces, and nephews. The doctors would try to harvest more stem cells after the new year rolled in.

Jennifer said, "We didn't know if we'd have another Christmas together. That took priority right then."

It was another great holiday for the kids. They were both showered with love, not to mention toys, clothes, and candy. But for mom and dad, there was a lot of stress under the surface.

"We knew we had to get back to Seattle and get those stem cells," Jennifer said. "We had the appointments set up, a three-month schedule of chemotherapy on the calendar, and a child with a tumor on his skull. It was all we could think about."

In between preparing meals, visiting friends, giving gifts, and all the other hectic, happy rituals of the season, Jarrett's parents had to book airline tickets, find a bigger apartment in Seattle, and make arrangements for someone to take care of their house and bills while they would be away.

Jarrett was to return to the Fred Hutchinson Cancer Research Center in mid-January. In the meantime, he had to have one chemo session in Kentucky so he would be on schedule. After the treatment and a few days before he was to go west again, there was another setback. The boy caught the flu.

Looking back, all Jennifer could say was that it was stupid not to delay the trip to Seattle. But that's 20/20 hindsight. At the time, it appeared their son could handle it, and she and Doug believed the clock was ticking.

Jennifer and Jarrett went to the Lexington airport as scheduled, with Doug planning to bring Claire along in a few days.

As soon as they got in the air, Jarrett started throwing up. It was as if the flu got up to speed as soon as the commuter plane did. It was just a fifteen-minute flight to Cincinnati and their connection. Jennifer told herself things would be better once they got on a bigger plane. The flight would be smoother and Jarrett could sleep. She just would not let him have anything to eat until they reached their destination.

It is a four-hour flight from Cincinnati to Seattle, but it seemed as if they would never get there. Jarrett threw up again about a half-hour into the second leg of their journey and was sick the rest of the way.

"I'm still mad at myself for not seeing how dumb it was to get on that second plane," Jennifer said. "He got so weak and dehydrated, he just slumped over in the seat. He was as pale as a ghost. The flight attendants took turns bringing him ice and cold cloths to put on his forehead."

The attendants also sat with Jarrett if Jennifer had to go to the restroom. It was obvious to everyone on board that this was a very sick little boy. Flying exacerbates dehydration. His mother tried to get her son to drink more water, but he just spit it back up.

On the other end, hospital volunteer John Hayes waited to meet the Mynears. The cancer clinic often paired out-of-state patients with local folks who could make their visit more comfortable.

"The man who was there to greet us had to come on board and carry Jarrett off the plane," Jennifer said. "It wasn't the introduction any of us had anticipated. But Jarrett was so limp I couldn't pick him up."

They didn't bother to check into their apartment or pull over to see any sights. The welcoming committee rushed Jarrett straight to the emergency room, where he was immediately hooked up to intravenous fluids.

"That's the worst of all the ordeals I'd been through," Jennifer said. "I was terrified. We were supposed to be there to get stem cells. Instead, Jarrett was admitted to the hospital with a violent and dangerous case of the flu.

"That's the only time I've seen him so sick he wouldn't talk to anyone. He withdrew and curled up into a ball. He wouldn't even reach for the phone when his dad was on the line."

Jennifer said she could actually hear crunching in Jarrett's lungs as he breathed. It sounded like gravel turning over in a storm drain.

The hospital booked Jarrett into a double room so his mother could stay with him. She would not have considered leaving, even if she would have had to sleep on the floor in a closet.

The next few days crept by, with Jennifer hanging on the edge of a nervous breakdown. Her husband and daughter were two thousand miles away, and her son right beside her seemed even more distant than that.

Jarrett spent the hours lying in bed, broken out in sweat, with IV tubes steadily dripping fluids into his body.

Jennifer made dozens of phone calls to Kentucky, talking to Doug, her friends, her mother, and Claire's babysitter—anyone who could help her pass the time. She knew it must be costing a fortune, but what was the price tag on her sanity? She felt she would surely go crazy if she didn't stay connected with the world outside Jarrett's hospital room.

When she wasn't on the phone, she worked crossword puzzles and thumbed through every old magazine in the waiting rooms in that section of the clinic. But there was no satisfaction in filling in the blanks or in reading what Hollywood starlet was back on the dating scene.

Sadness had taken up residence in her mind and body. Food didn't taste good, the TV sitcoms weren't funny, the mattress was hard, and the room was cold. She felt very old. It seemed the bright lights in her life had gone dim. Jarrett, whose spirit could usually outshine a lighthouse, was more like a nightlight now. There was still a glow about him, but right then he couldn't make the shadows disappear.

They were in a modern medical facility with an impeccable reputation. But to Jennifer, theirs was a room of gloom.

As she looked in the mirror over the sink in Jarrett's room, Jennifer knew she had to shake the blues. The dark circles under her eyes were a sign that she needed to be more concerned about her own health, both physical and mental.

"Jarrett's going to snap out of this flu in a few days," she told herself, "and he needs me to be strong and upbeat."

Jennifer gave herself a good talking-to and then picked up the phone again. She asked her mother if she could come join her in Seattle. Granny Jeanne was one step ahead of her daughter. She already had her suitcase packed.

After a week, Jarrett started to perk up a little. He was happy to see his granny and he wanted to know about other people back home.

He would sit up to watch television. He still liked Sesame Street and Barney, the purple dinosaur. And he paid attention to the local news. It helped him understand a little more about Seattle, the city outside his window.

He stayed groggy under heavy medication, but he was taking an interest in his surroundings. He was Curious George again, asking questions. The doctors thought Jarrett would make a great reporter someday. He already knew the five W's that reporters ask.

Who?

What?

Where?

When?

Why?

He didn't take notes, but he sure knew how to conduct an interview. His thirst for knowledge was back, keeping his mind active even when his body was too weak to stir.

The doctors decided they did not want to delay Jarrett's cancer treatment any longer. They needed to get more stem cells so they could go ahead with the stronger doses of chemo. The tumor had to be attacked—the sooner, the better.

As the preparations were being made, an anesthesiologist came in to meet the young patient, but he called Jennifer out into the hallway after being in the room for just a few minutes.

"He told me he couldn't believe anyone would think of putting this kid under," she said. "In his mind, Jarrett was still too weak. He said he didn't want to have any part in it."

Of course, that alarmed Jennifer. She already felt guilty about bringing her son to Seattle in his current condition. She didn't want to make another mistake.

On the other hand, the doctors were convinced Jarrett had seen the worst of the flu and that the stem cell procedure needed to be scheduled as soon as possible.

"I prayed a lot and decided I had to trust the doctors," she said.

When you are remodeling a house, you have to tear up to fix up. Things can sure be messy for a while but in the end, the results are worth it. Jarrett reminded his mother of a work in progress. Evidently, he had to get worse before he could get better.

Jennifer's decision was made all the more difficult by Jarrett's appearance.

"The bout with the flu had really taken a toll on him. He had lost so much weight, he was just skin and bones," she said. "At one point, he was on oxygen."

But she could tell he was getting stronger. Perhaps the heavy doses of antibiotics had done the trick. So she allowed the doctors to go ahead and put a temporary catheter under Jarrett's collarbone—an entry point for more needles. She would see how he handled that surgery before she gave the O.K. to allow another stem cell harvest.

When Jarrett woke up on the operating table, the rigid catheter was in place, looking like a straw sticking from his neck. He seemed to come through it just fine, so the next day the doctors again hooked up the drip tube and collected stem cells. This time, they got all they needed.

The doctors decided to delay the super-strong chemo treatment for a few more weeks. They wanted Jarrett to go home to Kentucky and get tougher. That's just what he did.

10

The Dream Factory

Before Jarrett headed back to Seattle in early March, he had another trip to make—up and down the aisles at Best Buy.

The nurses at UK had arranged for the little man to have a wish fulfilled by The Lexington Dream Factory, a nonprofit organization with the sole goal of spreading joy to seriously ill children.

Jarrett, now nearly six years old, had become quite an artist on his family's personal computer. He loved to make greeting cards and posters, and he had mastered the Paintbox program. But he never liked the way his works of art turned out when he ran them through the family's black-and-white dot matrix printer. He really wanted a color inkjet printer.

When he learned The Dream Factory wanted to let him pick out a printer at the electronics superstore, Jarrett perked up. The organization not only wanted him to get a printer, it had arranged a shopping spree. Jarrett was told he would be allowed to fill a shopping cart with any items he wanted that would help him pass the time in Seattle.

When the family showed up at Best Buy, it was greeted by three strangers: Terry Hagan, who was in charge of "dream procurement," The Dream Factory's past president Ralph Coldiron, and board member Leslie Beebe. They had a dolly waiting and told Jarrett to hop on and point the way. Jarrett knew right where the printers were, and off he went, like a tornado on four wheels.

It was the first time a television crew was made aware of Jarrett's condition. A videographer ran along behind the dolly, capturing the excitement and joy in Jarrett's face. A newspaper reporter kept close, too. The young man didn't mind the attention at all.

"We almost felt embarrassed that he wanted a printer," Jennifer said. "Doug and I were afraid it would look like we had asked him to get it for us. It didn't seem like the thing most kids would want, but it really was what Jarrett wanted most."

Only one would do—a high-resolution, top-of-the-line model by Epson. Terry Hagan worked for Lexmark, a Lexington-based company that specialized in printers, so he made a spirited effort to sway Jarrett away from his competitor.

"Look at all this one does," Terry said, holding up a printer that came off his employer's assembly line. "Wouldn't this be a better choice?"

But Jarrett had his mind made up.

"No offense, Mr. Hagan, but if you don't mind too much, I've already studied up on the Epson."

"He started talking about pixels and fonts and resolution," Terry said. "I couldn't believe how smart he was."

Terry picked up the printer Jarrett wanted and put it on the dolly.

"You know how much trouble I'd be in if my boss saw me do this?" Terry asked, jokingly. "Get me away from here. How would you like to go get some video games?"

"Really?" Jarrett squealed with delight. "I only planned to get a printer. Are you sure it's not too much?"

"We want you to have anything you'd like," Terry said. "It's all been taken care of. Don't worry about the price."

It didn't take long for Jarrett to select a handheld Sega Game Gear system. It was just the right size to take on an airplane.

"You'd better get some games to go with it," Terry said.

Jarrett picked out a Power Rangers game and a trendy one called "Sonic the Hedgehog." Terry held up four more.

"Do you think you'd like these too?"

Jarrett nodded in disbelief, and his new friend dropped them in the cart.

"We were amazed," Jennifer said. "We couldn't believe these people we didn't know cared that much about him."

Ralph Coldiron also tossed a hard plastic case onto the stack. In his head, he had figured up that the items in the cart would come to about $900. He didn't mind pushing it to a thousand.

"You'll need to protect that game system when you're traveling," he said. "Is there anything else you'd like?"

"No, thank you," Jarrett said. "You've given me too much."

The young television reporter asked Jarrett if she could have a few words with him on camera.

"O.K.," he said. "No problem."

As Terry was wheeling Jarrett toward the front of the store where the camera was being set up, Jarrett asked him to stop.

They were in the video aisle.

"Could I get one more thing?" he asked.

"Sure, what is it?"

"I'd like to get a movie for my sister."

Jarrett reached over to a shelf and took down a VHS tape decorated with a picture of Barney, the purple dinosaur.

"Claire would really like this."

The Dream Factory reps knew they hadn't gone wrong in selecting this kid for a treat. He was humble and grateful and unselfish. Deserving. Very deserving.

The reporter was surprised at how well Jarrett answered her questions. So were his parents. Although in the coming years, he would become a pro at television interviews, this was his first time in action. He told the reporter why he had wanted a printer, about the stem cell transplant he would receive in the coming weeks, and how he expected to be cured. And most of all, he kept saying how nice it was for the people at The Dream Factory to give him all these gifts.

"They're awesome," he said. "And they do this for other kids, too. I'm really glad I got to know them."

"He's a natural," the young lady said afterward.

Three months later, as Jarrett sat in the small apartment in Seattle recovering from the transplant, he took out a pen and paper. He had just celebrated his sixth birthday. Many of the cards he had received from friends and relatives contained money.

He took a $10 bill and stuffed it in an envelope, along with a note, scrawled in crayon.

> Dear Dream Factory,
> Last Feb. you gave me a shopping spree at Best Buy. I'm home from my transplant now. Use this money for someone else to get a dream come true. this is part of my birthday money.
> Your friend,
> Jarrett Mynear

Terry Hagan was astounded when he opened the letter and the money fell out. The Dream Factory had never had a child give back like that.

His mother said the organization taught Jarrett an important life lesson.

"He was really touched by what it had done for him, and he learned how neat it is to reach out and help others," she said.

An annual donation became a tradition for Jarrett. Ten dollars always came out of his birthday money.

"I'm sure $10 won't buy a dream, but every dollar helps," he said. "I want them to keep up the good work."

More examples of generosity were just around the corner. Jarrett would be on both the giving and the receiving ends.

11
Difficult Journey

Jarrett's parents had been deeply moved by The Dream Factory's acts of kindness. But the shopping spree also stirred some sadness in them.

"It was a validation that we may not come home from Seattle with our son," Jennifer said. "It was like he was being granted his *last* wish. We knew we were going into a horrible, life-threatening situation."

The return to Seattle came on March 5th, one day after the family celebrated Claire's second birthday. Special days are big for many families, but this foursome valued celebrations of life even more than most.

Right after the party, Jennifer finished packing the last of the things she thought she'd need out west—clothes, kitchen utensils, and toiletries. She also wanted to send a few toys and books that were familiar to her children. Jarrett made sure Raggedy Andy was going on the trip. They expected to be away from home at least four months.

"It was hard to think about being gone that long," she said. "We wanted to go quietly to the airport and just kind of slip out of town."

But on the morning of departure, more than a dozen friends and relatives showed up at the house to show their love and support. They helped the family carry bags to the car that was waiting for them, loaded Jarrett and Claire down with snacks and magazines to enjoy on the plane, and joked with Doug and Jennifer about how they were going to redecorate the house while they were gone.

Then, there was a scene that reminded you of the receiving line at a wedding. As the foursome headed to the car, each member had to stop for handshakes, hugs, and words of encouragement. Everyone was determined to get in his or her goodbyes.

As the car pulled away, the group of well-wishers stood in the driveway, waving like the Beverly Hillbillies did each week at the close of their show. Jennifer could tell Doug was tearing up, and she refused to look back again, knowing she would cry.

"I didn't want the kids to see us all weepy," she said. "We were trying to make this an adventure for them."

They held up pretty well for twenty minutes. Then, they went to their gate at the airport and found more friends waiting there.

As the plane lifted off, they looked down at the lush pastures of the Bluegrass, lined with white fences. Off in the distance, they could see the tall buildings that marked downtown Lexington. They were homesick already, but it was good to know there were people down there who would be praying for them and eagerly awaiting their return.

On this flight, there was a fifth passenger in the Mynear party, one who had never flown. Doug's mother, Mildred, insisted on going along to babysit with Claire for a week or so while her son and daughter-in-law went through another round of meetings with doctors.

Granny Mynear lived the simple life, having grown up without running water or indoor plumbing. She had never strayed far from the farm and had never been away from Paw for more than a day in their forty-four years of marriage. She found Lexington, with its 225,000 people, to be a big and sometimes scary city. She really couldn't imagine what Seattle must be like.

Doug's mother was as white as a sheet when the ground dropped out from under the plane. She didn't like one minute of the flight, but she was determined that if her grandson could go through all he was facing, she could endure the terror of flight.

"It was the sweetest thing," Jennifer said. "I can't tell you how special that was to us."

To Mildred, better known as Granny Mynear, it was just a simple way to help. To her family, it was a profound act of love.

12

A Kindred Spirit

Jarrett looked forward to a reunion on the West Coast. During his first trip to "The Hutch," as the Fred Hutchinson Center was often called, he made a new friend—one who was about forty-five years older than he was.

Just like Jarrett, Bob Hjort had crossed the country for a stem cell transplant. The native of Maine and his wife stayed in the same apartment building as the Mynears, and they often passed in the halls. Bob carried a portable IV bag with him everywhere he went.

"Looks like you and I are here for the same thing," Bob said to Jarrett as they each showed up at the cancer clinic to have their blood counts taken.

That was the opening Jarrett needed. He immediately began to ask the man questions about his cancer, his family, and his home in New England.

"They hit it off instantly," Jennifer said. "Bob and his wife Anita invited us to their apartment that night, and it was great to have some conversation with someone away from the hospital setting."

Bob and Anita had a Christmas tree in their apartment. That made their dwelling seem a little homier, even though the rooms were laid out exactly like the ones in the Mynears' unit. To Jarrett and Claire, a visit down the hall became like a trip to a relative's house, with different things to see and explore.

The families got together several times a week after that first visit. Within a few days, Anita hung stockings next to their tree. Two names were stitched in the fabric—

"Jarrett" and "Claire."

Bob taught Jarrett to play Hearts, and the man showed no mercy. He made it clear he wasn't going to relax the rules just because of Jarrett's age.

That made the boy all the more determined to claim victory. Sometimes, he would hide a card in his lap or under the tablecloth.

Bob would taunt him: "Cheat, cheat, never beat."

That was his chant over and over again. He would sing it out anytime Jarrett won, even when the boy hadn't cheated. It always made Jarrett smile.

During Jarrett's second trip to Seattle, Bob was one of the first people to get a smile out of Jarrett when the boy was suffering with the flu.

"Jarrett was lying there in bed, not really responding to anyone or anything," his mother recalled. "Then there was a tap outside the door."

It was Bob, carrying his IV bag and a deck of cards.

"Does anyone know where a man could find a good game of Hearts?"

Jarrett rolled over and his eyes lit up.

"You think you could beat me?" Jarrett asked, sitting up.

And the games resumed.

"Anita and I would sit and talk while the two of them played," Jennifer said. "I knew both of them were feeling miserable, but they kept each other going."

Bob also kept the family in stitches by recounting one of the unpleasant tasks of his chemotherapy. Doctors asked him to go through the distasteful routine of analyzing his own vomit and bowel movements. He had to fill out a form each time something came up or out. The form asked him to describe the texture and color of his "emissions."

"Where do they come up with these terms?" Bob asked, feigning indignation. "Foamy, creamy, soupy. Don't they know what puke looks like?"

"Eventually," Jennifer recalled while laughing, "he purchased a set of colored pencils and tried to match the colors in the margin of the form. We got quite a kick out of him trying to find out what two colors mixed together would best describe his stool. I guess after you've been through all we'd been through, you get a sick sense of humor."

If imitation is the sincerest form of flattery, then Jarrett paid Bob quite a compliment. Jennifer noticed one morning that Jarrett had filled out his own form after a trip to the bathroom. There were brown and yellow scribble marks in the margin, made by colored pencils.

When a third trip to Seattle rolled around, Jarrett didn't get to spend time with Bob. His card partner had his stem cell transplant a few days before Jarrett was scheduled to have one. There were complications, and Bob didn't live through it.

The Mynears kept that news from Jarrett for as long as they could, telling him that Bob just wasn't able to visit anymore.

Once again, Jarrett's parents were hit with the reality that this was a dangerous operation. Hit hard. They watched someone they had come to love slip away in an instant.

Bob had tried to cheat death.

"Cheat, cheat, never beat."

Their son would be the next person at The Hutch to lay his cards on the table. They prayed that for once he would be dealt a winning hand.

13

Transplant

Doug and Jennifer had never seen so much paperwork. Before the stem cell transplant could begin, they had to sign form after form, acknowledging they knew the risk their son was about to face.

"Basically, the papers said if we were lucky, our child would live," Jennifer said. "If we were really lucky, he would be rid of his cancer."

It was like buying a new, expensive product that came with no guarantee. No refunds, no exchanges.

"There were pages and pages of risks—everything from permanent brain damage to strokes and paralysis," his mother said. "We had to sign a statement that we understood this was a clinical trial. It spelled out all the positives and negatives, but the negatives seemed to go on and on.

"We read and read and searched the Internet. We talked to former transplant patients—anything and everything we could do to get more information."

But in the end, the choice was clear.

"We either had to do something aggressive or let him die."

Another week passed before the heavy chemo treatments could begin.

"The financial coordinators wouldn't even discuss proceeding until they found out if our insurance would pay," Jennifer said. The Mynears had been told that the minimum tally for this hospital stay would be $150,000.

Once the insurer gave the go-ahead, Jarrett began the hardest round of chemo he'd ever endured. This would be oral chemotherapy, requiring the five-year-old to take forty-two pills a day.

"Every time he turned around, it was time to take another pill," his mother said.

Besides the chemo pills, there were pills to prevent seizure, nausea, and bacterial infection.

Again, Jarrett was a trouper. He did what he was told, with little complaining.

At this point, his immune system had dropped to zero. That was the reason for this round of chemo—to completely kill the bone marrow.

His parents had to relearn how to take care of their son. As his primary caregivers, they had to go to classes on how to use a portable IV pump. Soon, many of his drugs would be administered at the apartment. And they had to learn about nutrition. Jarrett's eating habits had completely changed. The list of things he couldn't have was a lot longer than the list of things that were allowed.

"We got to a point where it was a goal to get him to eat twenty Cheerios a day," Jennifer said. "We would count out maybe five at breakfast, five at lunch and ten at dinner. His stomach was rejecting almost all food. We would try to add a few bites of fruit every now and then. Sometimes it stayed down, sometimes it didn't. Most of his nutrition came through a tube."

They had to become obsessive about germs and cleanliness. Everything in the apartment had to be scrubbed with Clorox every day—the counter tops, the cabinets, and floors. Laundry was an everyday chore as well.

"It was years until I could stand the smell of Clorox again," his mother said. "Our apartment smelled like a bleach factory."

During the first weeks in Seattle, Jarrett's parents liked to take him to the Seattle Arboretum. It was a beautiful place, like a peaceful Garden of Eden. But now, it was out of the question. Jarrett couldn't get dirty, couldn't breathe in pollen or be exposed to mold.

Two days after the last chemo treatment, he went into Swedish Hospital for the transplant. The hospital was partnered with The Hutch. The only thing his mother can remember about that morning is a feeling of nausea.

"I was a nervous wreck, and the room had the worst smell to it," she said. "You've never smelled anything like the preservatives they keep the stem cells in. It's a peach-colored liquid that drips into the patient's body. It's visually nauseating, too."

Half of the collected cells went into Jarrett's body and presumably straight to work, building back the marrow that had been killed off.

It was to be a seventeen-day hospital stay, with daily blood counts. The baby stem cells were growing up, turning into white cells and fighting infection. There was medical magic taking place inside a frail little boy.

Outside Jarrett's window, Seattle lived up to its reputation as a damp and rainy place. In Kentucky, some old-timers claim they know when rain's approaching simply by feeling it in their bones. Jarrett's parents had a feeling about the figurative weather, too.

Their intuition told them sunnier days were just ahead.

14

The Pink Ladies

The view from Jarrett's hospital room was like a postcard. Swedish Hospital stands on a hill overlooking Puget Sound. Jarrett's parents wanted to keep his mind strong, so they challenged him to imagine what was going in the world he could see outside his window.

He'd talk about the freighters coming in, trying to guess what they were hauling and what their destination would be. The large cranes that lifted cargo on and off the ships fascinated him. He dreamed up all kinds of scenarios about the men he saw walking along the shoreline and scurrying about the decks. Maybe some of them were pirates or spies or whalers.

Two days after his transplant, while he was gazing toward the harbor, a cart rolled into his room, pushed by two members of the hospital's auxiliary. The women looked quite cheery in their pink smocks.

Jarrett noticed right away that the cart was loaded down with toys.

"We didn't know anything about the toy program or the adult volunteers who made these visits," Jennifer said. "It was a nice surprise."

The ladies told Jarrett he could pick out something from the cart and keep it as their gift to him. He looked it over thoroughly, impressed with the selection of games, books, stuffed animals, and puzzles. He finally settled on a piece of string art—a picture printed on a piece of cardboard that he could weave yarn through to make a colorful display. It was something that could keep his mind and fingers busy.

As the volunteers turned to leave, Jarrett thanked them and asked when they would be back.

"Next Friday."

"I'll be here, too. See you then!"

In fact, Jarrett was there long enough to get three visits from "The Pink Ladies," as he called them. They were three visits that maybe took up fifteen minutes of Jarrett's life. But in those minutes, a seed was planted in the boy's fertile mind—one that would sprout three years later.

15

Recovery

The chemotherapy ended and radiation began. For the next eighteen days, doctors zapped Jarrett's skull to shrink the tumor. They had drawn marks on the top of his head to pinpoint the targets.

The stem cell transplant was really a two-part process. After a sixty-day recovery period, the other half of the collected cells would be returned to the boy's body.

"The doctors had a 'keep it coming' attitude," his mother said. "They wanted to do everything possible to make sure cancerous cells couldn't survive in his body."

So, they killed off the marrow once again, this time with radiation. Eight times in four days, Jarrett squeezed his body into a box, standing behind lead-lined shields to protect his lungs and liver as radiation penetrated his body.

Jennifer got another surprise at this time. The doctors told her Jarrett was doing so well that the next stem cell transplant could be done on an outpatient basis.

"They gave me IV bags filled with antibiotics and fluids to take to our apartment," she said. "It was somewhat disconcerting to think I'd now be responsible for his care, but I had been through training for it. It was good to think about spending less time in the hospital."

Around The Hutch, Jarrett's progress was all the buzz. He was a model patient and a perfect example of "everything going right." Someone from the public relations department approached Jennifer about bringing cameras to the apartment to make a training video for other parents. For one of the few times in her life, Jennifer said no to a request from Jarrett's medical team.

"I just had too much on my plate," she said. "Doug and Claire had gone back to Kentucky, and I was shuttling Jarrett back and forth for blood counts, changing IV bags, trying to fix meals, trying to keep the apartment germ-free, and so on, and so on. I just didn't feel like being in a video."

Those feelings of a nervous breakdown were coming on again, and Jennifer was determined not to crack.

She decided to rent a car. Their only transportation had been a van that made daily trips between the apartment building, the grocery, and the hospital.

Jennifer loaded Jarrett into the car, picked up a map, and headed out into the countryside, with the skyscrapers of Seattle in the rearview mirror.

"We needed to get away, even if just for two or three hours at a time," she said. "Jarrett couldn't get out and couldn't get in crowds, so we just became explorers in the front seat of a car. It did wonders for our morale. We took a road trip almost every afternoon."

One day, John Hayes, the hospital volunteer who had greeted the flu-stricken patient at the airport, came and said he wanted to show Jarrett one of his favorite places in Seattle. He drove the boy and his mother to a fishing pier near the Ballard Locks. Jarrett got out of the car and sat on a bench, watching the ships pass from one pool to the next.

"Are you getting hungry?" the volunteer asked, after an hour had passed.

Jarrett shook his head affirmatively. He was not hooked to IV nutrition, and he sure didn't want a handful of Cheerios.

"Let's try a place I think you'll like," the friend said. "Maybe you can handle a little *real* food."

And the Mynears were introduced to Chinook's seafood restaurant. As soon as they walked in, the smell of fried batter hit them like a letter from home.

Jarrett had a few bites of fish, three or four French fries, and half of a hush puppy.

"That really helped him snap out of his funk," Jennifer said. "Just like that, he was eating solid food again. We made several more trips to Chinook's in the days to come."

During one of the trips, the volunteer made a detour, driving Jarrett north on Aurora Avenue. They crossed a bridge and exited, making right turns until they were underneath the structure. Then Jarrett saw it. The Fremont Troll. It's one of the most popular, and strangest, art pieces in Seattle.

The large sculpture crouches under the bridge. Or, as locals say, it lurks. The Troll has a shiny hubcap for an eye and a long, stony beard. One hand grasps a real Volkswagen Beetle.

Jarrett wanted to get out of the car and get a closer look. He thought it was just about the neatest thing he had ever seen. He ambled over and looked up into the giant's face, awestruck.

Then more trolls appeared—real people in funny costumes with crooked walking sticks.

"Jarrett, we've been waiting for you," one of the trolls called out.

Other kids may have been scared. But not Jarrett. He was delighted the actors knew his name and went right up to shake their hands and play along with their silly skit.

"Do you like the Troll?" an actor asked.

Jarrett nodded.

"He likes you, too. He thinks you look delicious!"

Jarrett stepped back in mock horror, and everybody laughed. In fact, his laughter was constant for nearly an hour as he joked with the actors, tried on their robes, and forgot all about his cancer. There was some magic under that bridge, conjured up by the hospital volunteer, courtesy of the Fremont Arts Council.

The family lingered there, gawking and watching the other people who came by. Some came to take pictures. Others talked to the Troll and seemed to be expecting it to answer. A couple even left flowers, apparently as some kind of good luck ritual.

In the next few days, the Mynears discovered more about this part of the city. Fremont was the arts district, full of quirky shops run by aging hippies and hip new agers. The street corners were home to musicians and mimes, painters and puppeteers. It was a happy place for Jarrett.

And he always asked to go back under the bridge to see the Troll.

Susan Sever directed a school at The Hutch. She and two other teachers tutored children one on one. Most of their students were patients. Some were siblings of patients or the sons and daughters of patients.

She wasn't particularly fond of working with kindergartners. She usually tutored the kids of middle school age, preferring to teach geography, math, and science. She let another woman take care of beginning readers and kids who liked to finger paint.

But when Jarrett was there, the patient load was out of balance. There weren't many middle schoolers in the hospital, but the high school and grade school teachers were overloaded.

"I decided I could handle one kindergartner," Sever said.

The first time she walked into a hospital room to meet Jarrett, she wondered what she had gotten herself into.

"He was hyper," she said. "He was climbing all over the place and talking ninety miles a minute. When I told him I was there to teach him how to add and subtract numbers, he said, 'I already know that.' So, I said we would work on the alphabet. And he said he didn't need help with that either. He seemed like a know-it-all."

But Susan soon learned that Jarrett could back up his bragging. She was amazed at how much he already knew. And, like so many others, she was taken aback by his vocabulary.

"For such a tiny guy, he could sure use some huge words," she recalled.

Soon, she fell under Jarrett's spell and found herself spending more time in his room than she had ever planned.

"I found out how smart he was and how adorable he was," she said. "It was like we were on the same level, even though he was only five. Everything he said cracked me up. I had been ready to stay on the sidelines and see how quickly I could pass him off to another teacher. But after a couple of weeks, there was no way I was giving up my star pupil."

Susan had a friend whose daughter was about to be married. For a fun assignment, she decided to have Jarrett dictate some guidelines for a good marriage. The "handbook" was turned into a gift.

Jarrett's entries including the following advice:

1. Show you love someone by giving them presents.

2. Tell the other person when they do things you don't like.

3. If the other person starts an argument, tell them to stop.

4. If the other person doesn't stop, leave the room so you don't have to listen anymore.

Dr. Phil couldn't have given any better advice.

One day when Jarrett was in a makeshift classroom set up at the hospital, a deliveryman came to door with some items for the school. Jarrett played in the far end of the room as Susan signed for the package.

The deliveryman seemed unsettled to be there and asked Susan in a low voice if all the kids there had cancer.

"Not all of them," she said, as Jarrett got up and bounced over to the doorway. "But this one does. Look at his bald head."

She patted his shiny scalp playfully. The man still looked uncomfortable.

"Actually," Jarrett spoke up ("actually" had become his favorite word), "I've had cancer since I was two. It was in my leg, and they cut it off. Now, it's in my skull but they can't cut my head off!"

Then he let out a loud, hysterical laugh.

"That man backed out of the room quickly and *actually* seemed frightened," Susan said.

Jarrett and Susan joked the rest of the day about how it would be if the hospital cut kids' heads off. There'd be little monsters roaming the halls, holding their hats in their hands because they wouldn't know what to do with them. It was silly talk—the kind that keeps your mind off the bad stuff.

Susan's philosophy was that tutoring provides hope.

"School is a future-oriented thing," she said. "If you instill in a child that he needs to learn his multiplication tables, the implication is that he's going to live."

She would read lesson plans to children as they drew their last breaths because she believed in staying positive until the end.

When Jarrett was five, she honestly did not think she would get to spend many more months with him. But in the years that followed, she made annual trips to Kentucky to see her all-time favorite student.

"I packed my bags many times, thinking I'd have to go back to Lexington for a funeral," she said. "Jennifer would tell me that Jarrett had relapsed. I'd brace myself and get really sad. Then, in no time, he would rise again and be as vibrant and mischievous as ever."

Susan said she has not been a "super-spiritual" person, but "there's something special that kept Jarrett hanging on. His life had a reason."

In 1999, Susan was diagnosed with non-Hodgkin's lymphoma. She told Jarrett about it on her annual visit to see him.

"He gave me the greatest pep talk and told me how the bone marrow aspiration I was scheduled for wouldn't really hurt that much," she said. "He told me it was O.K. to be sad but only for a little while. Then he said you have to get on with life."

Spring passed and summer arrived in Seattle. Now, homesickness really took over. Jennifer wanted to tend to her garden back in Kentucky and eat hamburgers fixed on the grill behind their house. She missed Bluegrass traditions, such as attending the horse races at the Keeneland track. Jarrett was ready to go back and play outside with his friends and show off his newfound video game skills. That Sega system from The Dream Factory had gotten a workout. Jarrett had reached the highest level of play on every game he owned.

"He used to sit in the clinic and get so excited with those games that his hands and legs would twitch," Jennifer laughed. "One nurse asked if he ever put the thing down. It was his 'clinic thing.' He never touched it at the apartment."

Mother and son set a goal. They hoped to get back to Kentucky in time for Jennifer's birthday, July 11th. She made the airplane reservations.

"The doctors said that wasn't the way things should be handled," Jennifer said.

"But they had faith in our doctors in Kentucky and knew that we lived close to a hospital. So they agreed that they would try to approve Jarrett's release by our pre-determined return date."

Jennifer began sending things back to Kentucky. They had accumulated so much stuff that it cost $200 in shipping charges. Some things they could leave behind, but not the three toys Jarrett had received from The Pink Ladies. They were good luck charms.

16
Saying Thanks

They got home on their schedule. Jarrett didn't really get to roam the fields and run the ridges like he had hoped.

His parents had to be strict about visitors and going places. They had been told it would take about a year after the transplant for Jarrett's immune system to build back up.

But he was home, in his own room. Best of all, they felt like a family again. Discussions took place across the dinner table instead of through a phone line.

Jarrett had been home just a couple of weeks when his friends at The Dream Factory came calling again, this time to give him a job.

They wanted him to be their special guest speaker at their annual gala, an elegant affair where many of the region's movers and shakers made big pledges to help pay for "dreams." It was to be a dinner and dance in the ballroom of the Marriott Griffin Gate resort hotel, followed by silent and live auctions.

"We didn't know that meant hundreds of people in the same room," his mother said, admitting naiveté. "He was supposed to be in isolation. But he wanted to do it, so we said he could."

Jarrett's appearance was to be a surprise to the people in the audience. The organization's president, Terry DeLuca, kept him out of sight until it was time to begin the program from the podium.

Jennifer and Doug sat at a table near the front of the banquet hall, feeling intimidated and underdressed. The room was full of men in tuxedos and women in beautiful evening gowns. The Mynears had scanned the bid sheets on the tables spread with silent auction items and could see that money was no object to a lot of these people.

Jennifer wore a nice dress, but it certainly was not a ball gown, and Doug had on a gray suit and tie. They wondered if they really stuck out as badly as they felt they did. And, nervously, they wondered what might come out of Jarrett's mouth when he got behind the microphone.

Their apprehension vanished quickly. When Terry began to introduce Jarrett, she choked up. She told the crowd about Jarrett's $10 donation and how he had been the first child to send money back to the organization that had helped fulfill scores of dreams.

"He's here tonight so you can see where your money goes," she said. "He'd like to speak to all of the donors. Please welcome Jarrett Mynear."

Jarrett strode to the stage, looking sharp in his tiny rented tux and red bow tie.

The crowd rose to its feet in unison, and the applause was loud and long. Doug and Jennifer stood, too, overwhelmed by the reception their son was receiving.

When the crowd settled down, Jarrett pulled a short and simple speech out of his pants pocket.

"I don't know how to thank you enough," he said. "Your gifts helped keep me get through a lot of lonely days. Terry asked me if I'd read my letter to you, so here goes."

He then read from another piece of paper, the thank-you note he had sent earlier that year—the one that was wrapped around a $10 bill.

Again, the crowd erupted in approval. Jennifer looked around and saw a lot of people wiping tears from their eyes. Then she realized. These people weren't here because they had big bank accounts. They were here because they had big hearts.

After the speech, Jarrett's parents couldn't keep up with their son.

"He was working the room like a politician," she said. "Everyone was asking to have a word with him—asking us to send him over to their table next."

He posed for pictures, signed autographs, and got his cheeks pinched by well-meaning ladies more than a few times.

As the evening progressed, a band took the stage and the dancing began. The lead singer called Jarrett up to the stage and handed him the microphone. The next thing Doug and Jennifer knew, their son was singing along to the Bob Seger classic "Old Time Rock and Roll."

There was the squeaky voice amplified. His parents just shook their heads. Apparently Jarrett had been talking to more people than they realized. They don't know when he had a word with the band, but somehow he'd had a conversation that had won him a solo in the spotlight.

It wasn't exactly beautiful music, but it was as uplifting as any hymn. It was the sound of a happy heart, and it filled the room.

17

The Silly Season

Jarrett started first grade in January 1996, again running about a half term behind everyone else in his class. As he had done in preschool, on his first day, he explained his medical condition to his fellow students. He took a sharpened pencil and stabbed it into his right leg.

Some of the kids gasped.

Jarrett laughed.

"See, it's not real, and some of you didn't even know it," he said. "I'm not handicapped."

"The teachers and principal were very sensitive to Jarrett's needs," Jennifer said. "The school let me draw up a letter asking the other parents to please keep their children at home if there were any signs of illness—the flu, chickenpox, mumps or measles. They were all cooperative and understanding."

Jarrett turned seven in April, finished first grade in May, and had a summer to remember.

He went swimming almost every day. He discovered new video games. He teased his sister. Two or three times a week, one of his adult friends from The Dream Factory or church or the neighborhood took Jarrett out to eat or to a movie or baseball game.

"He had a better social life than we did," Jennifer said. "He was as comfortable in a room full of adults as he was on the playground."

Jarrett was due for a checkup at The Hutch. The doctors there like to see their patients on an annual basis for a progress report. The family planned their return for mid-June, on purpose. The Fremont Arts Council—all those people who played trolls for Jarrett under the bridge—had invited them to be in the Solstice Parade. They weren't really sure what they were getting into, but it sounded like fun.

Jarrett's exam at The Hutch went off without a hitch. So they stayed in Seattle a few extra days, awaiting the Saturday closest to the first day of summer—parade day.

"The Solstice Parade is unlike anything you've ever seen," Doug said. "There are only two rules for entrants. You can do anything you want as long as it's not in a motorized vehicle. All the floats had to be human-powered. And there could be no advertising."

The arts council reserved a place for the Mynears on a large pull cart made up to look like a pirate's ship. The theme was Peter Pan. Jarrett was given a pirate's costume, complete with a plastic sword and golden necklaces. Claire was dressed up as Tinkerbell. Jennifer decided she would just walk along beside the float, out of costume. Doug was glad of that; the fewer things on the float, the better.

"I found out I was there to play horse," he said. "They needed me to help pull the thing, and it was heavy. There were four other guys there to help, but a couple of them spent more time dancing in the street."

Tens of thousands of people lined the street. The event was outrageous—sort of a northwestern Mardi Gras—a way for people in a rainy climate to welcome the season of sunshine. They passed street performers and fire-eaters, drag queens and belly dancers. A gay-themed Wizard of Oz float told them Dorothy wasn't in Kansas anymore. And the Mynears sure weren't in Kentucky.

Jarrett looked like a king, albeit a scruffy one with a fake beard and eye patch, as he waved to the crowds and took in the wonders.

"At one point, a group of bicyclists whisked by us on the street," Doug said. "They were all nude. I looked back at Jennifer, and she looked horrified. Then we looked up at Jarrett. He was grinning ear to ear."

"Oh, well," Jennifer said later. "What could we do about it? You can't control streakers, and it gave Jarrett another good story to tell when he got back home."

18
"Go, Jarrett, Go"

The Dream Factory gala rolled around again, and Jarrett wasn't about to miss it. His parents tried to tell him it was an adult affair and his invitation last year had been an exception.

"Remember," his mother said, "you were the only kid in the room."

But deep down Jarrett believed he'd be invited back. He loved The Dream Factory, and he had sent them another $10 in the past year. Didn't all donors get an invitation?

He was right, of course. When Doug and Jennifer's invitation arrived in the mail, the handwritten addition was clear: "Please bring Jarrett. We look forward to seeing him again."

Jarrett was especially interested in the silent auction. The year before, he had paid close attention to all the items spread out on tables awaiting the highest bidders—neat things such as computer scanners, cell phones, boom boxes, and calculators. He'd like to try his hand at naming his own price for some neat gadgets.

Granny Mynear had given him $40 just for that purpose. It nearly burned a hole in his pocket. As soon as they arrived, he began to peruse the treasures up for bid.

Just like the year before, Doug and Jennifer soon found themselves on the edge of the room watching Jarrett get the star treatment. Again, he was doing the shake-and-howdy "nice to meet you" routine.

At one point, they saw their son sitting on top of a Sea-Doo personal watercraft that was to be auctioned off. Moments later, they scanned the room again and saw him in the driver's seat of a go-cart, brightly painted with Valvoline Oil logos and slogans.

His name was the first one to be written on the bid sheet for the go-cart. He'd gladly spend the whole forty for the shiny machine.

"He was having the time of his life," Jennifer said. "After we'd been there awhile, someone came over and asked, 'Do you know who Jarrett's talking to now?'"

They didn't recognize the handsome gentleman who was showing Jarrett around the auction items.

"That's Ron Turner," they were told. "He's one of the most successful businessmen here."

Turner was a developer and the chief operating officer of Amteck, an electrical contracting company that did business all over the world. He had invested wisely, and his home was one of the city's showiest. Each Christmas, he and his wife Linda covered their all-white mansion with thousands of miniature lights and invited sick and underprivileged children in to see Santa Claus. Ron put on the beard and took each child on his lap to hear their wishes. The parties always concluded with the kids being loaded into a white horse-drawn carriage for rides through the neighborhood.

To Jarrett, he was just another nice guy in the room—someone he was glad to get to know.

An hour before the bidding was to end on the silent auction, while Jarrett was still shaking hands and posing for pictures, board member Ralph Coldiron came over to the table to whisper something to Doug and Jennifer.

"Mr. Turner wants to know if it's O. K. for him to buy the go-cart for Jarrett," Ralph said.

"We were blown away," Jennifer said. "What were we supposed to say? If we said 'no' it would look like we were being mean. We knew the money would go to The Dream Factory, which was a great thing. Ralph said Mr. Turner sincerely wanted to give it to Jarrett. In fact, he was already working behind the scenes, encouraging other potential buyers to make sure he got the last bid."

"I could tell by watching him that he really wanted it," Ron said later. "I really didn't care how high the bidding got."

The clock approached 11 P.M., way past Jarrett's bedtime. But Doug and Jennifer let him stay to see how the auction would turn out.

The emcee began a countdown to officially close the bidding.

"Three . . . two . . . one . . . all done."

The last bid on the clipboard next to the go-cart was by Ron Turner for $900—nearly three times what it was worth. But he had purposely placed the bid out of reach.

Everyone still in the room knew Ron didn't plan to ride around in the thing, and they watched as he made his way over to Jarrett's table.

"Congratulations, Jarrett," he said, extending his hand. "Looks like you get the go-cart."

"That's not possible," Jarrett said. "I only bid $40. I know it went for a lot more than that."

"The best bid wins," Ron said. "Your bid wasn't the highest one, but it was the best one."

Jarrett was overjoyed and couldn't find the words to thank Mr. Turner enough. All the way home that night he was thinking about that colorful go-cart. Gala organizers had promised to deliver it the next day. Jarrett would be waiting at the crack of dawn.

The next morning, a van pulled into the driveway at the Mynears' home. Jarrett heard the noise and ran to the window. He saw two men unloading his dream machine.

Jarrett rushed out and claimed his prize, eager to take it for a test drive. But that would have to wait. The car needed some modifications. Ron had thought of that, too. He had sent word that he would be out to measure little Jarrett and check out the position of the controls, the gas pedals, and the brake.

So for two days, Jarrett spent several hours just sitting in the cart, making racecar noises with his mouth and whipping the steering wheel right and left. At last, on the third day after the auction, Ron showed up with his two sons, took Jarrett's measurements, and loaded the go-cart into a pickup truck.

"Don't worry," he told Jarrett. "We'll bring it back in a couple days."

Over the years, Ron and Linda Turner got to know the Mynears quite well. They always invited the family to their Christmas party, as well as company picnics at Amteck. The Turners often invited Jarrett out to eat at some of his favorite restaurants because they loved to hear him talk about life.

"You never heard about his problems," Ron said. "He never complained about anything. He fueled my heart. He had more hope than anyone I knew and no fear. Being with him was like being in church. It made me thank God for how fortunate I was. I needed him around to help me keep my focus on what was important. A visit with the Pope couldn't have had more impact on me."

When the go-cart came back, it was custom-fit for Jarrett. His name was painted on the side right where the driver would sit. And Claire's name decorated the back panel. She was listed as "Pit Crew."

Jarrett got in, started up the engine, let his foot off the brake and headed off through the yard.

"Watch out for the bushes!" his mom called out.

Jarrett swerved a little to the right, then a little to the left, and eventually got the thing straightened out. Jennifer thought her son was going to give her a heart attack with this new "toy." But, she remembered all the months when Jarrett's mode of transportation was a wheelchair or a gurney—when his daily route was from a hospital room to an examining table.

"Go, Jarrett, go!" she yelled, hugging Doug and laughing as their little Mario Andretti did donuts in the driveway.

19
After Summer Comes the Fall

Jarrett started second grade in the fall and all signs were that he was bouncing back from his cancer just fine.

Then September came. The Mynears had come to dread the ninth month of the year. It was at a September football game when Jarrett first alerted his family to his "hurts" as a toddler. And it was September of his kindergarten year when he was diagnosed for the second time with Ewing's sarcoma.

As the calendar turned again, so did their luck. Jennifer discovered another lump on Jarrett's head.

"He kept telling us he bumped his head on the swing set," she said. "But the bruise on his head wasn't in the same spot as the bump."

Jarrett seemed to be searching for any explanation he could find. He didn't want to believe it could be cancer again. Neither did his parents.

"Mom, I'm sure it's where the swing hit me," he insisted. "You worry too much."

But the lump was quite visible, the size of a pea. It doubled in size overnight as he slept. And that was that. There would be no arguments or second-guessing. His mother took him straight to the hospital.

The doctors performed a fine needle aspirate, which means they sucked cells from the lump through a hollow needle. The results showed the cells were cancerous.

Again, the calls and consultations began between the doctors at UK, the Mayo Clinic, and The Hutch.

The bottom line was the stem cell transplant had not worked, at least not permanently. Although it had seemed to build Jarrett's strength and keep the cancer at bay for a while, it had not killed off every trace of the disease.

The doctors suggested yet another round of chemotherapy.

Doug and Jennifer were told Ewing's sarcoma was considered a "smart cancer." The disease learns to adapt to chemotherapy. Treatment that works for a while can soon become ineffective. It's sort of like the flu. The vaccines are ever changing as new strains turn up and the body adapts to the shots. Or think of cockroaches. You can spray a house with pesticides and get rid of the bugs for a while. But over time, they can become resistant to the chemicals and can thrive despite your efforts to kill them. You have to find different, stronger sprays. The "cancer bugs" in Jarrett's system just hadn't been exterminated.

"We now knew Ewing's was just not going to go away for good," Jennifer said.

So, the next round of chemo was different than all the previous ones. The doctors tried new combinations of pills and poisons. Jarrett was pulled out of school and Jennifer officially resigned from teaching.

By this time, the Mynears had another situation to complicate their lives. Claire had been diagnosed with ADHD, Attention-Deficit Hyperactivity Disorder. She also suffered from sensory motor integration dysfunction. From about the time she was three, they noticed she had trouble following instructions and her speech was slurred.

Although her body was healthy, her mind was not developing as it should. She had all the symptoms you associate with a "hyper" child—a short attention span, bursts of high energy and a low tolerance for frustration. She could be an extremely loving, outgoing child one minute and shy and reclusive the next.

Her parents were determined to help her get the disorders under control. That meant another child with appointments to make, medicine to take and obstacles to shake, as they shuttled her to meetings with occupational and speech therapists.

This family was burning the candle at both ends and in the middle. To borrow a cliché, at times they truly didn't know which end was up.

The routine continued through the fall and winter. By summer, the Mynears had taken on a whole new attitude about Jarrett's lot in life.

"We had let the cancer rule our lives long enough," Jennifer said. "During each round of treatment before, we kept a tight rein on him. We decided to stop being so protective and isolating of Jarrett. If someone wanted to take him somewhere, within reason, we let him go. If visitors wanted to come by, we made them feel welcome."

The family took advantage of every opportunity to go swimming and hiking. They made many trips to Nicholas County so Jarrett could trek in the woods around Granny and Paw Mynears' farm. And they also decided that summer to send Jarrett to camp.

It was a decision they would never regret.

20

Indian Summer Camp

Many people had tried to sell the Mynears on the idea of sending their son to camp. Parents of other children with cancer, doctors, nurses, and friends from the American Cancer Society all told them how uplifting the experience could be. Kids could go at the age of seven, but Doug and Jennifer didn't believe Jarrett was strong enough for it then.

But during the summer of his eighth year—the summer they decided to let Jarrett live life to its fullest—they let him sign up for Indian Summer Camp. Jarrett had seen the brochures and was more than ready for a week of "roughing it."

Doug and Jennifer drove their son to the camp, an hour away in Estill County. Raggedy Andy was right there with him in the back seat.

"I suggested he might want to tuck Andy away," Jennifer said, concerned other kids would tease him about having a doll.

"He said, 'I don't care what they think. Andy is my de-stresser and he goes where I go.'"

Other the years, Jennifer had replaced the ribbon on Andy's shirt many times because Jarrett had worn it to threads by nervously rubbing it between his fingers while waiting for doctors and nurses to come into his room. And, despite her apprehension, no one ever made fun of Raggedy Andy—not at camp or even later when Jarrett was in middle school.

The last three miles of the journey were down a narrow gravel road, where tree branches formed a tunnel and kudzu vines dropped down from utility poles. Jennifer and Doug wondered if they were taking their son into a wilderness full of spiders, snakes, poisonous plants, and swollen streams.

Jarrett hoped so. As he pressed his nose to the car window and waited for a glimpse of his weeklong home away from home, Jarrett envisioned himself as an Indiana Jones sort of adventurer.

"It would be the longest he had ever been away from us," Jennifer said. "We were worried, but yet we knew many of the doctors and nurses who would be there to take care of him. They were ones he had already worked with. We trusted them, so we had to learn to let go a little."

They felt better when the road opened up into a clearing and they got their first glimpse of the campsite. The first thing Jarrett saw was the swimming pool. He'd be in that thing first chance he got.

There were rows of cabins and a large central building. The Mynears saw a volleyball net, a pit for campfires, and a lake lined with canoes. The lawns were neatly mowed and the sun dropped light on the miniature village, making it look like an oasis in the middle of nowhere.

And, for Jarrett, the best sight of all was other kids—dozens of them, laughing and running around like they didn't have a care in the world. Many of them were bald, some were missing limbs and a couple of them were in wheelchairs. But if you closed your eyes and listened to their laughter and their chatter, you could have been at any camp in the country. Sure this was "cancer camp," but it was about living, not about coddling kids and concentrating on their troubles. There would be no pep talks or speeches about coping with the disease. As much as possible, the camp's counselors aimed to ignore individual disabilities. Everyone here was in the same boat and, for this week, that boat was pulling up anchor and setting sail.

Jennifer and Doug met the counselors, chatted with some of the other parents and took a good look around. With dusk approaching, they headed back up the gravel road in their car, telling themselves and each other that Jarrett would be just fine. It had been good to see all those kids they had come to know in hospitals at someplace more pleasant.

"But truthfully, we worried every night," Jennifer said. "This was before cell phones were prevalent. I would worry when I left the house to run an errand or go to the store that someone from the camp would be trying to reach us. I gave them about twenty phone numbers. I was like an old mother hen."

The camp director called the Mynears midway through the week. When the phone rang, Jennifer immediately feared something was wrong.

But the director was calling only to check in and tell them Jarrett was having a wonderful time.

"He told us that even though Jarrett was one of the youngest kids there, he had become somewhat of a leader," Jennifer said. "He said Jarrett was the voice of reason when some of the other kids wanted to get into things beyond their abilities."

And he said the young man was willing to try any activity the counselors had planned. He excelled at the arts and crafts, he was among the first to volunteer for any game, and some of the girls appeared to have a crush on him. That made Jennifer smile. She could picture her talkative son getting tongue-tied around the young ladies. And she knew he would be trying to hide in a corner on the last night of camp when a dance was on the agenda.

The counselors were especially happy that Jarrett had tackled a thirty-foot climbing wall. As he pulled himself to the top, his prosthesis came unattached and tumbled to the ground.

"Oospy," Jarrett shouted. "Look out below!"

Everyone laughed.

People often brag that they can beat their competitors with one arm tied behind their back. Jarrett could do it with one leg lying on the ground.

The week went quickly for Jarrett.

"I had a blast," he told me. "I was the only kid there with Ewing's, I think. But I really didn't know what the other kids had. We didn't talk about it. That was one of the nicest things about it. No one felt sorry for us."

Every day, even though it rained a lot, the campers went to the pool. Swimming was Jarrett's favorite pastime. To visitors, the pool deck could be an unsettling sight at first. The chain link fence was lined with artificial limbs, as the kids bobbed around in the water unhindered by manmade devices. Some of the kids wore caps to keep from getting sunburned on the top of their bald heads.

What else did the kids do? Anything you can name as a camp activity probably occurred there. They made beaded necklaces and tie-dyed tee shirts. They played hide and seek in the woods, fished in a pond, and played "horse" on the basketball court. They took up archery and practiced self-defense. And at night, they sang songs around the campfire and told ghost stories after the lights went out.

For Jarrett, the last day was the best of all. It was a day when his skill at video games would serve him well in a real life battle—a battle of precision and wits where no one got hurt. The campers had been told they could end the week with "the water fight to end all water fights." And they came armed with their super-soakers.

The campers formed a circle in an open field, holding their weapons, with their hearts racing. They had teased each other all week.

"Wait 'til the water fight. You're the first one I'm going to soak."

"That's what you think. I'll get you first."

"The wetter the better. Bring it on!"

When the director gave the signal, the fury began. With squeals of delight, the campers ran around for more than an hour, soaking each other from top to bottom. The counselors got in on it too and the kids ganged up on them.

"Some firefighters were there with one of their trucks," Jarrett recalled. "They had a big hose we could use to refill our guns. And they let the kids take turns using the hose to shoot streams of water into the crowd."

There were no winners in the battle. Everyone was equally drenched and equally delighted. It looked as if that same boat they were all in had capsized. But everyone came up gasping for air. Actually, they were breathing in life, deeply, and drinking in all that was good about childhood.

In later years, the water fights ceased. The camp moved to a new location and new operators decided to ban anything that resembled weapons or warfare. Most of the parents thought it was a shame. On one hand, they could understand the argument. But the kids missed the battles, and no one saw them as violent or aggressive. It was good, clean fun and by the end of the week, the campers needed cleansing.

"I think that first week, Jarrett had had one bath," Jennifer laughed. "He came back with rashes and lots of dirt under his nails and behind the ears. The water battle had made a muddy field even messier. The counselors just kind of went with the flow."

Their son, who had spent much of his life in pristine hospital rooms and apartments sterilized with Clorox, had been allowed to get down and dirty. It seemed right. He had wrestled germs and handled worms. In other words, he was allowed to be a normal eight-year-old boy.

Jarrett never missed camp after that.

"Going back the next year was an automatic," his mother said.

Several of his counselors kept in touch with him throughout the years, and his doctors were good about working his chemotherapy schedules around camp.

Once a patient turns 18, he can no longer attend Indian Summer Camp unless he or she comes back as a counselor. Jarrett decided the first year to make that a goal.

"I plan to go keep going there as long as I live," Jarrett said. "It's been one of the highlights of my life and if I can give back by being a counselor, I'll definitely do it."

He said he would even dance with the girls.

21

Promotion

Jarrett attended third grade for two weeks. And for once, September didn't bring bad news.

"His teacher came to us and said our goals for Jarrett were being squashed," his mother said.

"What do you mean?"

"I mean he's so far ahead of the other kids, he's not getting the social interaction you want him to get in school," the teacher said. "We have him working in a corner on other projects that are more at his level. He's working by himself too much."

The teacher and the principal wanted the Mynears to consider letting Jarrett skip ahead to the fourth grade.

"That shocked us," Doug said. "We knew Jarrett was smart for his age, but he had been out of formal schooling so much that we really didn't think he was that advanced."

His parents were also concerned about his size.

"He was so much smaller than the other kids, and this would put him in middle school early," Jennifer said. "We really had to think about it.

"We worried about the maturity factor, but the teacher assured us that wouldn't be a problem. Jarrett had always made friends easily and already knew a lot of the kids in the fourth grade, so that wasn't a big issue."

They certainly didn't want to hold Jarrett back, and they could tell that he was bored with his homework assignments. So they let him move up a grade.

"It was the right thing to do," his mother realized later. "It gave him a sense of belonging."

Jarrett loved going to school. For him, it was a privilege.

"He thought other kids took it for granted, and that bothered him," Jennifer said.

"When he was out for a chemo treatment or because a flu bug was going around, other kids would say to him that they wished they could stay out of school for a week at a time."

Jarrett bristled at that.

"He'd say, 'No, you don't know what you're saying. Given the choice between school and chemo, I'll take school any day.'"

Fourth grade was Jarrett's first complete year of elementary school. He was there on the first day and he was there on the last day. He took part in a full cycle of lessons and a full cycle of extracurricular activities, from fall festivals to spring field trips.

But shortly after he turned nine in April, Jennifer's maternal antennas went up again.

"I started seeing symptoms of exhaustion," she said. "He really seemed to be tired and draggy. It was all he could do to get through the day. He would come home from school and just collapse on the couch. It was not like him at all."

He was still going in for blood counts, and they always hovered just above the transfusion level. His platelet count was low, and he bled easily.

She talked to his doctors about what was happening, and they agreed his blood cell counts should have been building up more by that time.

"They said his marrow was tired. It was just taking him longer to regroup this time around after his latest chemo treatments. They said I needed to relax and be patient. He would bounce back."

But Jennifer's instincts told her it was something more. Jarrett was developing spider veins on his shoulders and back. That just could not be normal, she told herself.

She was right.

22

An Open Book

This is the part of Jarrett's life story that Jennifer had trouble sharing with anyone. It was weird. Mystical even. She was concerned it made her sound crazy.

She was cleaning the house one day and noticed one of their reference books on the shelf—one of the many medical manuals they had acquired over the years. She took the book down and dropped it on the floor.

"I did that just to remind myself to check it out later, after I was finished with the housework," she said. "I thought with it lying out I'd have to stumble over it and force myself to do a little research."

She did indeed stumble onto something.

When she came back to the book, it was lying open to a page that described a condition called myelodysplasia.

"I had never heard of it before," she said, "but I was immediately drawn to the article."

The symptoms it described matched what she was seeing in Jarrett—lethargy, spider veins, and low blood counts. The disease was defined as a pre-leukemia condition that develops when the bone marrow wears out. It was typically a disease of elderly people.

"I had the strangest feeling that I was supposed to see that article," Jennifer said. "It was like a guardian angel led me to it. I thought maybe even my dead father had a hand in it.

"I know that sounds loony, but that's how I felt."

She asked Jarrett's doctors if he could have myelodysplasia. They said it was a possibility, but a remote one.

Doug had to leave for business on a Monday morning, the same day as Jarrett's next doctor's appointment. His company assigned him to Italy to work on a reverse osmosis water treatment plant at a U.S. naval base. It was just the second time his employer had sent him overseas.

Jennifer dropped her husband off at the airport on her way to taking Jarrett to the doctor's office. He kissed his wife and son goodbye, promising to return in a week with some souvenirs from Naples.

At the clinic, Jennifer again asked about the articles she had read.

"They were respectful of my instincts and said they would do a bone marrow biopsy to test for a blood virus or something that could be causing the low counts. They thought a biopsy would rule out myelodysplasia."

Once again, they stuck a large needle in Jarrett's hip and drew out marrow. Then mother and son went home to wait for the results.

Doug called as soon as he got settled into his hotel room in Naples, just to let his family know he had arrived safely and to give out the phone numbers where he could be reached. There was a six-hour time difference. It was late at night in Italy, but still early evening in Kentucky.

"I told him about the bone marrow biopsy," Jennifer said. "I could hear concern in his voice. He tends to be more optimistic than I am, and he hadn't really thought the doctors would see a need to do more tests."

"Let me know the minute you hear anything," Doug said. "I won't be able to sleep until I know something."

As soon as Jennifer hung up from talking to Doug, the phone rang again. It was Jarrett's doctor. Bad news traveled through the telephone line like a bolt of lightning. If anyone else had been in the room, they would have seen Jennifer's complexion turn instantly pale, her posture slump, and they would have heard her voice become a quivering whisper.

The voice on the other end confirmed her fears. Jarrett did indeed have myelodysplasia. His bloodstream contained leukemia cells—the result of all the chemotherapy that had ravaged his body over the past seven years. Now Jarrett was battling two diseases.

"What do we do now?" she managed to ask the doctor, as she felt her knees go weak.

He said there were really only two options. The first was palliative care, which basically means just doing your best to make the patient comfortable until the disease takes over. The other was a bone marrow transplant.

The message was loud and clear. Jarrett was at death's door. The doctor didn't put it in those words, but that was understood.

The diagnosis came on the eighth anniversary of the death of Jennifer's father.

"I couldn't have felt sadder," she said. "I was truly almost ready to give up, sort of thinking enough was enough. I didn't want to face my son again, who was feeling miserable, and tell him he had another disease and needed another risky treatment."

She told herself that maybe it was selfish to try to keep him alive. She loved him more than words could tell, but was it fair to put him through so much? If God wanted Jarrett so badly, maybe they should let Him have him. The thoughts swirled through her mind, and she would get mad at herself for even thinking of giving up. Then, she would get mad when she thought her decision might prolong Jarrett's pain. She needed Doug to help her think it through.

She tried to call his hotel room, but she couldn't get an operator who spoke English. She didn't know anyone who spoke Italian who could put in a call for her. She tried several times, but each time she hit a brick language barrier. So Jennifer sat by the phone, knowing Doug would call her as soon as he could.

On the other side of the Atlantic Ocean, Doug too had trouble getting an operator who could help him make a connection. After several frustrating attempts, he went to bed. He tossed and turned and stared at the clock.

The next morning he went ahead to work. It was 8 A.M. in Naples but just 2 A.M. in Kentucky. He didn't want to disturb his family in the middle of their night. And he assumed Jennifer hadn't heard back from the hospital yet.

Late that afternoon, Naples time, Doug did get to a phone and got through to his wife. When he got the news, his reaction was the same as Jennifer's. He too turned pale and weak, feeling as if he had been run over by a steamroller.

"I immediately said I had to get home," Doug said. "There were two other guys from the company on the trip. They could take up my part of the presentation."

He told Jennifer he would be on the first flight he could get out of Naples. The company would help him make the arrangements.

But before he hung up, he left Jennifer with some words that helped her put things in focus.

"We've been through all these years together and not once has Jarrett shown any signs of being a quitter," Doug told his wife. "He'll be the one to tell us when it's time to give up. We'll have a long honest talk with him and see what he wants to do."

They were both pretty sure they knew what Jarrett's answer would be.

23

A Perfect Match

To even consider a transplant, doctors would have to find a donor—someone whose bone marrow matched Jarrett's tissue type.

Bone marrow is a soft fatty tissue that produces blood cells. Marrow damaged by chemotherapy and radiation cannot produce enough white cells to fight infection.

The doctors told Jennifer parents rarely provide a marrow match for a child. Brothers and sisters match somewhat more often, but it is usually a stranger who provides the marrow for a transplant. Still, they wanted Jennifer and Claire to be tested right away. Doug would be tested as soon as he returned from Italy.

There are several stages of testing. Jennifer did not match even in the first stage. Claire did.

"Claire was physically drawn into this," Jennifer said. "That worried us. Doug and I would have gladly given anything—arms, legs, organs. But we didn't know if Claire could handle it."

Doug got in late Thursday, weary from travel. He went through the blood testing the next morning, and he was not a match either. But more good news came back concerning Claire. Every stage of the testing showed her to be a perfect match. Doctors called it the best case scenario. The Mynears weren't so sure about that.

"We were concerned about the emotional trauma for her, not just the physical trauma," Jennifer said. She hadn't liked it at all when they drew blood for the tests, and her hyperactivity was still a concern. Although she had grown up in and around hospitals, she had never been a patient.

That night at home, Doug and Jennifer had that long, honest talk with Jarrett. They told their nine-year-old son just what they knew about myelodysplasia. They told him it was the reason he felt tired all the time, why he bruised easily, and why he sometimes bled without any reason. They told him it could develop into leukemia, a full-blown blood disease.

"We tried to remind him what a transplant meant," Jennifer said. "It meant intensive chemotherapy, a long hospital stay and months of recovery. We asked him if he was up for it."

"I don't have much of a choice," Jarrett said emphatically. "It's either do it or lie down and die, and I'm not going to lie down and die."

His parents looked at each other knowingly. It was the answer they had expected, certainly the one they wanted.

Next Doug and Jennifer went to Claire and tried to explain to her what was ahead. Jarrett too had expressed concern about drawing his little sister into the process. But Jennifer sensed something as she talked to Claire. The girl seemed to take pride in the fact that she was the only one in the family who could help Jarrett now. During all those previous trips to hospitals, she had been helpless to do anything for her big brother. In all her hyperactivity over the years, she always seemed to understand that she had to take it easy around Jarrett. She could not jump on him or play too roughly with him. When he needed his sleep, she knew to tiptoe around him. She never seemed jealous of all the attention he got. But now the attention was on her. She could literally save her brother's life.

She told her parents earnestly and lovingly that she would let the doctors stick needles in her if it would help Jarrett.

"I'll do whatever they need me to do," Claire said. Her parents couldn't have known she would take it this well. Did she really understand? She was just six years old. They believed she knew enough to realize they wouldn't ask her to do it if it weren't important. They hugged her and told her how special she was.

The next battle was with the insurance company. Bone marrow transplants are not always covered. Each individual case is considered separately. The company had already paid more than $700,000 for Jarrett's care over the years. It didn't approve new procedures without a lot of scrutiny. This transplant could cost anywhere from $200,000 to $400,000.

"We didn't have time for them to drag their feet," Jennifer said. "Leukemia cells called blasts were developing in his bloodstream, and the numbers were increasing each week while we were waiting to see if insurance would pay."

His blast level hovered around twelve to fourteen percent. The Mynears were told if it reached twenty-one percent, the doctors would not do a transplant. It would be too late than. Leukemia would win out.

The Mynears had to decide where to go, should the transplant be approved. Usually, a patient would go back to where he or she had their original treatments. But the family was reluctant to pack up and relocate to Seattle again.

Dr. Greg Hale, a pediatric oncologist at UK's Markey Cancer Center, helped the Mynears with their decision.

"He personally delivered research articles to us at our house," Jennifer said. "He talked with us over coffee about the procedure and answered any questions we had. He said he had the equipment at Markey to do the transplant. He had done the procedure for patients with myelodysplasia, and he was willing to do it again."

They asked Jarrett what he thought.

"These doctors know me here," he said. "They care about me and know what I need. I'd like to stay here close to my family and friends."

"Although Jarrett liked Seattle, he also equated it with the worst time of his life," Doug said. "He didn't want to go there again unless it was to be for a vacation."

That settled it. Once the insurance company said O.K., the transplant was scheduled for mid-August at the Markey Cancer Center in Lexington.

By the time the procedure was approved, Jarrett's blast level had reached seventeen percent. Once again Jarrett had raced the clock and come in under the wire.

Transplant day came August 12, 1998. Granny Jeanne stayed in Jarrett's room. Doug and Jennifer went into pre-op with Claire. When Dr. Hale was ready, Claire was wheeled into the operating room with her Sesame Street slippers peeking out from under the sheet. The only smile in the group came from the Muppet character Elmo at the ends of each of her feet.

The doctors gave her an anesthetic, and in a matter of minutes, she fell into a deep sleep. The surgeons bored into Claire's pelvis in two places, using hollow needles to suck the marrow from her bones.

Fluid was drawn from her body into a plastic container. It was then taken away to be filtered and treated.

In a room down the hall, Jarrett was eating tacos and watching television. His immune system was at zero. The marrow in his bones had been completely killed. But the casual observer would not have known he was at a crossroads in his life. He seemed at peace, without a care in the world.

Late in the afternoon, the doctors came into his room. They had the IV bags, which were like presents from his sister. They contained the gift of life.

The tubes were connected to Jarrett's catheter, and the fluid began to flow into his body. It was naturally transported back into the bone cavities where it was expected to grow quickly to replace the old bone marrow.

Claire woke up and tried to roll over. A sharp pain shot through her back. She was wrapped around the waist by a large pressure bandage. There was an intravenous needle stuck in her hand, the IV pump was churning—all things she had seen Jarrett experience. She began to cry.

"Honey," her mother said. "It's over. You'll be all right. Jarrett has some of your bone marrow now. We're so proud of you."

Claire slept peacefully through the night and was eager to go home first thing the next morning. She left the cancer center by skipping out the front door, with no need for painkillers. The Mynears realized they had more than one resilient child.

24

Jarrett Gets an Idea

As Jarrett recovered from his bone marrow transplant, he spent another thirty-eight days in isolation at the University of Kentucky's Markey Cancer Center. But his hospital room looked like a playhouse.

Get well cards covered two walls from ceiling to floor. His mother had brought tacky putty to hang them all where Jarrett could see them. He enjoyed looking at the "wall of love" with its funny pictures, jokes, and notes of encouragement.

A friend also supplied their son with a laptop computer so he could get e-mail and play online games. And one corner of the room was piled high with stuffed animals, books, plastic trucks, and puzzles. The Nintendo 64 system seldom sat silent.

Jarrett couldn't leave the room, but plenty of people came to him. It seemed as if the stream of visitors was nonstop—relatives, neighbors, friends, and parents of other children who were patients in the hospital. And there were several doctors, nurses, and hospital aides who counted themselves among Jarrett's newfound friends. They too popped into the room whenever possible. It was good to see a cheerful child who made them laugh.

The phone rang several times an hour with people wanting to let Jarrett know they were thinking about him.

"It was amazing," Jennifer said. "It really kept him going. He wanted to be here now instead of in Seattle. This was where most of his friends and family were."

Kathy Tabb, an American Cancer Society volunteer who had come to know Jennifer through support groups, became a daily visitor to Jarrett's room.

"We bonded," Kathy said. "I just wanted to relieve some of the strain on Jennifer, but I didn't know what I'd talk to a kid about. But when he found out I was a survivor of ovarian cancer, he just started talking about things that were familiar to me—doctors we both knew, articles we had read, things we did to pass time in the hospital. It was like talking to someone my own age."

Kathy brought daily gifts to Jarrett, mostly junk items she picked up at a dollar store. She always wrapped them and kept him guessing what would come next.

He liked to blow bubbles and squirt water pistols. She gave him lots of things to foster his mischievousness.

"Once I took him a can of silly string, and he sprayed it all over his bald head," she said. "He always had the nurses in stitches."

One day, during a rare moment without visitors or phone calls, Jennifer talked to Jarrett about how fortunate he was to have so many people who loved him and wanted to be near him.

"Jarrett had noticed the rest of the ward seemed quiet compared to his room," said Jennifer. "We talked about the fact that some of the kids didn't have a lot of visitors and didn't get many cards and gifts."

Jennifer stepped out of the room for a few minutes to get a cup of coffee. And in those moments of solitude, Jarrett's mind went to work.

"I thought somebody should do something for those other kids," Jarrett said.

And even though he was just nine years old, Jarrett decided he should be that somebody.

When his mother came back into the room, Jarrett sat up in bed and told her he had an idea. He reminded her about The Pink Ladies in Seattle and how much he enjoyed the gifts they brought around once a week. And he mentioned the trinkets Kathy brought him each day.

"Couldn't we get some toys together and start a cart here?" he asked, with such sincerity it almost made his mother cry.

"I was stunned that he came up with that idea," Jennifer said. "He had four catheters hanging out of his chest and was under heavy medication. He was in bad shape, and he was thinking of someone else."

Jennifer is the first to admit her son was not always the angel he appeared to be. He could be temperamental and hardheaded, like all preteens. But at that moment, she could almost see a halo over his head.

"After the initial shock of him coming up with that suggestion considering the shape he was in, I told him we'd talk to his dad about it," she said.

"I certainly didn't want to discourage it, but I wasn't sure how much thought he had given it."

Because of their experiences with The Dream Factory, Jennifer knew they had contacts who would probably help them get a gift-giving drive together.

"I thought we might get enough toys to go around the hospital once or twice, and then Jarrett would probably lose interest," she said.

"The children's hospital has fifty beds, so I told Jarrett we would need fifty toys. He had a couple of duplicate toys he said he'd be willing to give away, but he didn't want to give out anything that had been used or opened. He wanted the kids to have new toys, not hand-me-downs. That was hospital policy, anyway."

In the weeks that followed, Jarrett was released from the cancer ward, but he wasn't able to go to school. Doctors feared he would pick up some childhood disease from such close contact with large numbers of children. Even a common cold could be a setback to all the progress he was making.

A teacher came to the house for two hours a week for homebound lessons, but that wasn't nearly enough instruction time to be acceptable to Jarrett's parents. Jennifer, with her background in teaching, insisted on spending many hours with her son in educational pursuits.

One of those pursuits became the toy cart. Jarrett talked about it all the time. He wanted to make it happen as soon as possible, so his mother told him to work out a business plan.

Jarrett wrote out a list of goals and objectives. It was much more ambitious than what his mother had in mind. It soon became obvious Jarrett wanted the toy cart to be a permanent fixture at the hospital, not just something that came around once a year like Christmas.

He wrote letters to the administrators at the hospital, seeking their blessing. Then he made a list of people and businesses that might donate. And he went straight to the top, writing letters to the big department store chains such as Toys "R" Us, Walmart and K-Mart. In fact, every store in Lexington's largest mall got a request for money, toys, or both. Jarrett sent about a hundred letters in all.

Even though the basic request was a form letter, Jarrett signed a personal note attached to each mailing.

Word spread among the family's many friends. Ralph Coldiron, The Dream Factory's past president, was also on the board of the children's hospital. He was instrumental in making sure all the influential people he knew would help make Jarrett's endeavor a reality.

"I saw Jarrett one day in the hall of the clinic," Ralph recalled. "He had a mask on his face and wasn't looking too well. The first thing he said to me was 'Ralph, I want to start a business. Will you help me?'"

Ralph heard Jarrett's idea and loved it. He told his young friend he would contact the head of the Children's Hospital Fund to get the ball rolling.

"He was a ball of fire. He knew exactly what he wanted to do."

But admittedly, Ralph didn't act on it right away.

"About a week later, Jennifer called me to ask about it. I asked her how serious Jarrett was, and she said it was all he was talking about. I got on it that same day."

Kathy Tabb remembers the first time Jarrett told her about it.

"He said he didn't want a lot of adults getting involved because they would just have a lot of meetings and waste a lot of time," she said. "That cracked me up. Did he have the business world figured out or what? I've used that quote many times."

The young man also decided to put a little twist on the name of his project. He changed the name from "toy cart" to "joy cart." He said it was about spreading happiness.

"He totally came up with the name," his mother said. "We had to admit 'Jarrett's Joy Cart' had a nice ring to it."

His family decided to keep the items small. They asked for the toys to be valued at no more than $10. They thought it would be easier to stock the cart that way and prevent one child from getting a video game console while another got a box of crayons. Uneven giving might defeat the purpose of spreading joy and harmony.

"Everyone has things they donate to, and I thought we might have to dig into our own pockets to make this thing happen," Jennifer said. "I didn't want to disappoint Jarrett if it didn't work."

That was wasted worry. In just a week after the letters went out, Jarrett started getting positive replies and, even better, checks. From the initial mailing, he got a twenty-eight percent response rate. Marketing experts will tell you to be pleased if you get five percent.

The folks at the children's hospital were caught up in the excitement, too. Once the public relations staff found out The Joy Cart had enough donations to make an initial run, it arranged a news conference.

"I wanted to put it off," Jennifer said, still not sure if the donors were committed long-term. "But once the date was set, there was no stalling."

March 23, 1999, fell during the middle of the NCAA basketball tournament, so local news crews were spread thin. The Mynears were told not to expect a large turnout at the news conference. But the public relations department had received a few phone calls and knew the cart would receive some coverage.

"When we walked into that room, I was blown away," Jennifer said. "There was a room full of reporters and four or five video cameras."

There were nearly a dozen microphones on the table, bearing the logos of all the local television affiliates—Fox, ABC, CBS and NBC—and several radio stations. Bright lights were set up in each corner of the room, and every other person seated there had a notebook or tape recorder in his or her lap.

"Jarrett had been interviewed one-on-one before to help promote The Dream Factory," Jennifer said, "but he had never faced a barrage like this."

A hospital spokesman made a couple of remarks to start the news conference, then he turned things over to Jarrett. The nine-year-old calmly outlined how he got the idea for the cart and how the cart would work, and he read off names of people who had donated toys or money. Then he took questions, expertly describing his cancer and the operations he had been through. He had the audience in the palm of his hand.

"I remember Doug and I watching the interviews," Jennifer said. "He didn't miss a beat, and the media people were fascinated. We had no idea he would be that eloquent in a crowd."

When a reporter asked Jarrett's parents if they had anything to add, they were at a loss for words. Jarrett had just about covered it all.

One of Jarrett's friends from the hospital was ushered into the room for the ceremonial first toy pick from the cart. Little Jordan was a quiet child, not at all outgoing like Jarrett. But Jarrett insisted his buddy do the honors.

The patient looked over the hospital cart at the end of the conference table and pondered for a minute.

"Take anything you'd like," Jarrett prodded.

That was not an easy decision for a child. The cart was overflowing with books, puzzles, action figures, games, cars and trucks, spongy balls and stuffed lions, tigers and bears.

Jordan chose a beanie baby, formed in the shape of "Lucky," the horse mascot of the local hockey team, the Kentucky Thoroughblades.

Cameras began to flash, and TV crews moved in close to capture his expression. Jordan stood there mesmerized. Jarrett walked in beside him, with a smile brighter than any light provided by the media.

Next, Jarrett got behind the cart and said it was time to make the rounds. The cameras were welcome to follow.

With a hop and a limp, off he went, steering the cart down the hallway from room to room. It was like that shopping cart you always seem to get at the grocery store. One wheel seemed to have a mind of its own. Jarrett joked about his driving skills, and the reporters laughed almost every step of the way.

In each room, Jarrett stopped to make his pitch to the child who was making the hospital home for now.

"You can have anything you want," he said. "It's free. Take your time. Get something good."

He sounded like a carnival barker hocking his wares:

"Step right up . . . have I got a deal for you . . ."

When a little girl automatically reached for a beanie baby, Jarrett made sure it was what she really wanted, pointing out some other "neat things" on the bottom shelf of the cart. And when a boy said he would like to have a book, Jarrett reached under a stack and pulled out *Treasure Island*.

"I'd recommend this one," he said. "Robert Louis Stevenson is a really good writer."

Again, the members of the media laughed. Not only was Jarrett a pint-sized Santa Claus, he was a literary critic, too.

After each room had been visited and the journalists were long gone, Jennifer took Jarrett to lunch at KFC.

"We were in high spirits, chatting about the turnout and all that had happened," Jennifer said. "All of a sudden, a firefighter came over to our table and said he wanted to shake Jarrett's hand.

"He said, 'You're Jarrett Mynear, aren't you?'"

The pair couldn't believe the instant recognition. The firefighter had just heard a story about The Joy Cart on the radio, and Jarrett's distinctive voice gave away his identity in the restaurant.

The fireman told Jarrett to keep up the good work.

Celebrity was something the Mynears would have to get used to. Soon, Jarrett couldn't go anywhere in central Kentucky without being recognized.

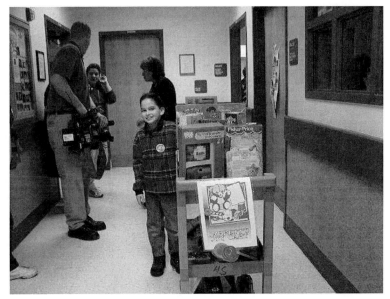

Jarrett prepares to make a Tuesday night run with The Joy Cart

25

My Turn

Even though that news conference was well attended and received numerous mentions in the local media, I couldn't help but think Jarrett's Joy Cart deserved more in-depth coverage.

I arranged to go to the hospital a month later—after the cart had made a couple of runs—for a progress report. Although Jarrett was charming in the first stories, it was a staged setting. I wanted to talk to him one-on-one, without four other cameras and stacks of microphones stuck in his face.

My videographer Jeff Knight and I pulled into the loading zone in front of the University of Kentucky Hospital just as the Mynears were unloading their van.

We quickly made our introductions. Jarrett said he already knew who I was. He was often allowed to stay up long enough to watch at least part of the *Fox 56 Ten O'clock News*, the show I anchor each weeknight.

He called me to the back of the van and excitedly began to show me all the new things he had to add to his cart that week. His sister Claire also ran right up to me like she had known me forever. I could tell she was excited about the project, too. She had been riding in the back of a van that looked like Santa's sleigh.

A month after its inaugural run, the cart wasn't running low of supplies. Quite the contrary. New donations were coming in every day. In fact, Jarrett's mother told me she would be ashamed to show me the family room at their house right then.

"There's no room to walk," she said. "We're going to have to find some storage space."

The hospital's child life specialist, Mary Kane, showed up to greet the family at the curb with three carts. The family tried to sort the toys into age-appropriate categories as they loaded the carts. One held toys for the patients under three. Another one was for those between four and ten. Then there was a cart for the older kids.

I told Jarrett we would like to just follow him and watch him do his thing.

"For now, try to pretend we're not here," I told him, knowing that was not a realistic request.

So Jarrett started to push the blue cart down the sidewalk, heading for the entrance to the children's wing. The cart had a loud, squeaky wheel. I remembered thinking this must seem like the ice cream truck to the kids inside. They can hear it coming and know it is full of treats.

"Oopsy," Jarrett said. I heard a bang and noticed he had struck the concrete wall as he was steering around the videographer.

"You might want to stay back a little bit," he told Jeff. "I've been known to run over people."

Upstairs, the public relations folks had already scouted the rooms in which it was O.K. for us to record. Several parents had signed permission slips, agreeing to allow their child to be televised.

In the first room we met a little boy named Cameron. The lights were off, making the room seem dreary. He was connected to some type of monitor.

Jeff and I went in first so we could witness Jarrett's entrance. I tried to make small talk with Cameron, but he didn't speak. He just looked at us with suspicion. But when Jarrett came in and said he was giving away toys, Cameron sat up and fixed his eyes on the cart.

Jarrett steered it as close to Cameron's bed as he could and began to hold up items.

"Just let me know when you see something you want."

The boy pointed to a plastic dinosaur and Jarrett handed it to him. Cameron's grandmother, who was sitting in a chair by the door, thanked Jarrett.

"That's so nice of you," she said.

"Oh, you're welcome," said Jarrett, as he wheeled the noisy cart back out the door. "See you next time."

There came that lump in my throat again. Outwardly, two boys couldn't have been more opposite. Jarrett was outgoing and energetic. Cameron was quiet and shy. But I knew they shared a silent bond— knowledge of what it means to be cooped up in a hospital, feeling pain and facing uncertainty.

It was a three-minute visit. As we left that room, I looked back and noticed Cameron had propped the dinosaur next to another one he had no doubt received on Jarrett's last visit. I wondered how big his collection would grow. How many weeks would he be there for visits from The Joy Cart?

In other rooms, Jarrett met other children who knew him by name. Undoubtedly, every other Tuesday was a day they all had marked on their calendars. Jennifer's mother had already told me privately they would soon start running the cart on a weekly basis. There were enough donations to make that possible. Wouldn't that be exciting news for the long-term patients?

"How are you feeling this week, Christopher?" Jarrett said cheerfully to a five-year-old boy.

"Better," said Christopher.

"I brought you a truck like you wanted," Jarrett said.

Christopher gave Jarrett a big smile and slapped his hand with a high five.

We went into another room where a boy fixed his eyes on the cart and fell into deep thought. He looked over every toy three and four times. Jarrett tried his best to help with the decision, pulling out games and books from the bottom shelf and demonstrating how certain magical contraptions worked.

"How about this denim dog?" Jarrett asked. "It comes with a marker and you can get people to sign it."

"I just can't make up my mind," the boy said.

"Do you like sports?" Jarrett tried again. "Here's a sticker book about baseball."

Frankly, I was beginning to lose patience with the patient. We had a news story to shoot, and Jeff had all the video we could possibly use in that room. But Jarrett never got in a hurry.

At last, the boy settled on a large poster of a monster that came with colored markers. That ought to keep him busy for a while, I thought. But he may have finished scribbling on it before we got to the next room.

"It's overwhelming for some kids," Jarrett told us. "They're afraid they'll only get one chance to pick a toy, and they don't want to blow it. But the truth is, I'll see most of them again."

After we had gone to five rooms—all of the ones we had permission to visit—I asked Jarrett's father to grant me an interview in a conference room. He agreed to do that while Jennifer and Jarrett continued distributing toys to the other forty-five rooms on the floor.

Doug told me the story of how Jarrett was diagnosed and a condensed version of all he had been through. He related the words of the child psychologist at the Mayo Clinic, the one who told them Jarrett would be the strong one through all this.

"It's true," he said. "He has indeed been the one to get us through."

Then it was Jarrett's turn. He came into the room and allowed Jeff to run a wireless microphone up his shirt. I knew immediately I could ask this nine-year-old the same kind of questions I would ask an adult. Interviewing children can be one of the most challenging things a reporter ever has to do. But talking to Jarrett was easy. Knowing where to start was the hard part.

He told me all about The Pink Ladies, the business plan he devised to get donations, and the response he had received since the first news reports aired a month earlier.

"What's the main reason you're doing this?" I asked.

"Well," Jarrett said. "It's not really about the toys. It's about giving the kids something to look forward to.

"We went into a room the last time I was here and my dad told me the girl in there hadn't been out of bed for four days," Jarrett said.

"But she got out of bed and walked across the room to pick out a toy. That made me feel so great to know that I was able to do something that good."

My eyes got watery again. I noticed the public relations assistant who was sitting in the back of the room was choking back tears, too.

I asked Jarrett if he had any advice for other children who found themselves spending a lot of time in the hospital.

"Well," he said in that high-pitched voice, "I'd tell them that they'll have some bad days, but not everything that happens in here is bad. They'll meet some good doctors, and they should ask them lots of questions. They're here to help you feel better."

I asked Jarrett how long he planned to continue the project.

"As long as I'm able, I plan to keep The Joy Cart rolling," he answered cheerfully. "And if I ever can't do it, I hope someone will keep it going in my name. I want it to be my legacy."

How many nine-year-olds know the meaning of the word *legacy?* Jarrett had a keen understanding that he had already defeated the odds. He seemed at peace with the notion that a long life is not a guarantee for any of us. *Carpe diem.*

The story wrote itself. I didn't have to do much narration. Jarrett's words and actions said more than I could ever say in a script. Jeff's video was excellent.

After I introduced the piece from the news desk a couple of nights later, I again watched the reaction in the studio. The man behind the teleprompter took out a handkerchief, removed his glasses, and wiped his eyes.

This boy was touching people's hearts. That was a gift greater than anything he could stock on his cart.

Months later, that story won a regional Emmy. My name is on the trophy, but Jarrett made the magic. As I accepted the award, I told the audience it was one of the greatest pleasures of my career to share Jarrett's story. I meant it then and I mean it now.

26

A National Audience

A member of our production department at the television station told me he would like to send videotape of my story to one of his former girlfriends. Making copies of stories is one of the time-consuming tasks we are always being asked to do in my business.

"Sure, I'd be glad to make you a dub," I told Dave Blair. "I'll try to get it to you in a week or two." I think I made some joke about being used to help him get back together with an old flame.

But he urged me to do it as soon as possible. He told me his ex was on the staff of *The Rosie O'Donnell Show*.

"This is just the kind of guest she likes to book," Dave said. "I know they would want to have him on the show."

Dave was one of those behind-the-scenes people whom I had seen get choked up viewing my story. I respected him a lot. But I wasn't sure about sending Jarrett's story off to a national production company. Maybe his parents wouldn't want to be bothered with it.

But the more I thought about it, the more I realized Dave was right. This was a touching story that could reach a national audience. I knew Jarrett could talk to anybody. He wouldn't be intimidated by the experience if the show's producers did indeed want to have him as a guest. I decided to let Dave send the tape and see what, if anything, would happen.

In less than a week, New York was on the line to our newsroom. The producers of *The Rosie O'Donnell Show* told us they had booked Jarrett to be on the show in just two days, and they wanted all the raw tape we could provide. Our station didn't air Rosie's show in the Lexington market, and giving out raw tape was against company policy, especially if it was going to go to a program aired by one of our competitors. But the news director was himself a member of The Dream Factory board. He was willing to make an exception in this case.

He knew the exposure could bring in donations, and he believed Jarrett's Joy Cart definitely deserved to keep going.

Doug and Jennifer were reluctant to accept the invitation at first. The producers called on Monday and wanted Jarrett to fly to New York on Tuesday, which would be his third day at another session of Indian Summer Camp. Jarrett loved camp and looked forward to it all year.

"If it were up to me, I would've said we'd be right there," Jennifer said. "But I wasn't sure how Jarrett would feel about it. Rosie's assistant promised they would fly Jarrett back to Kentucky as soon as the show was over, meaning he would only have to miss one night in his cabin."

The show was about to go on hiatus for the summer, and the Mynears were told it just wasn't possible to hold the taping for another week.

So Jennifer called the camp and got one of the nurses on the line.

"Jarrett was off playing somewhere, so I didn't get to tell him directly about the invitation," she said. "The nurse got all excited and began screaming to other people there in the room that Jarrett was going to be on *The Rosie O'Donnell Show*.

"I said 'Wait a minute. See if Jarrett wants to do it. I won't tell them to make the reservations unless he says he's O.K. with leaving camp.'"

The nurse found Jarrett, relayed the message, and called Jennifer back in a matter of minutes.

"His exact words were 'I'm going to New York!'" the nurse said.

The word spread quickly around camp and the other kids were maybe even more excited than Jarrett.

Jarrett hadn't seen *The Rosie O'Donnell Show*, but he knew who she was. He had seen her host the *Kids' Choice Awards* on Nickelodeon.

So, the whirlwind trip was on. Doug and Jennifer packed an overnight bag for each of them and one for Jarrett. They made arrangements for a babysitter to keep Claire. They picked Jarrett up at camp, which had moved that year to Shelby County, about halfway between Lexington and Louisville. All the other campers came out to give him a sendoff.

"Make sure you mention us on TV," more than one friend told him.

The Mynears made the forty-five-minute drive to the Louisville airport and flew to New York for a date with the "big time."

Like all first-time visitors to New York, Jarrett was amazed. The buildings just seemed to go on forever as he watched from the airplane window.

"There are a lot of people down there," he thought. "And a lot of them are going to see me on TV."

A stretch limousine met them at the airport and took them straight to a large hotel near the NBC Studios, where the show would be broadcast at 10 o'clock the next morning. It would be shown live in New York and on taped delay to the rest of the nation.

Once they got settled, the family set out to get dinner. But they had one stop to make first. Jarrett had heard about FAO Schwarz, one of the world's premiere toy stores. A lot of people know it from the movie *Big*. It's where Tom Hanks played "Heart and Soul" with his feet by jumping on a giant electronic keyboard.

The taxi pulled up and Jarrett gazed up at the building as if it were the gates of Heaven. But there was a sign on the door: *Closed for a Private Party.*

Jarrett's heart sank. He was an avid fan of *Star Wars* and *Episode One: The Phantom Menace* had just been released. He had read about a *Star Wars* display at the toy store, complete with movie props and costumes. And, as a kid who loved Lego blocks, he was determined to locate a *Star Wars* play set he had been unable to find in Kentucky. He was sure there was one inside that huge store, but now he would never know.

Rosie's staff had arranged reservations at Mars 2112, a kid-friendly theme restaurant. Visitors got to the dining area by riding a flight simulator that conjures up images of outer space. The idea was to feel you had been transported to a futuristic Red Planet. Robots danced about the room and the menu listed such things as the Crater Burger and Cosmic Cheesecake.

"It was neat place," Jennifer said. "We were all fascinated by it."

But despite the fun atmosphere, Jarrett was a little quieter than usual. His family wasn't sure if it was because of the disappointment about the closed store or because he was thinking about the next day's broadcast. They knew they had butterflies in their stomachs, and they weren't the ones who would be on stage.

When the Mynears got to the studio the next morning, staffers from Rosie's show met them at the front door. Everyone knew right away who they were and made the family feel right at home. If people in New York were supposed to be rude and uncaring, you sure couldn't have proven it at the NBC Studios that morning. They were ushered to a dressing room backstage. The star on the door displayed the name of Cheri O'Teri, a member of the *Saturday Night Live* ensemble.

"Wow," thought Jennifer. "This really is where the celebrities hang out."

A large fruit basket sat on a table in the room along with a tray of croissants. The refrigerator was stocked with juice, soft drinks, and bottled water. It was "the royal treatment."

Production assistants subtly moved in and out of the room, quizzing Jarrett for tidbits of information. It was like a reverse police interrogation. Anything he said could and would be used in his favor.

"They were good at what they do," said Jarrett's mother. "They would slip notes to each other and leave, I guess to make notes for the show and phone calls."

They found out about Jarrett's fascination with *Star Wars* and about the missed opportunity to visit FAO Schwarz. The Mynears would find out later the conversation was more than small talk.

Jarrett was told how he was to enter the stage, where he would sit, and how he should address the cameras. One woman powdered his face. He wasn't sure about that.

He also learned he would be in good company this day. The other guests on the roster were CBS news anchor Dan Rather, singer/actress Jennifer Lopez, and Michele Williams of the television drama *Dawson's Creek*. June Lockhart would also be appearing with the latest incarnation of Lassie.

Each star was in a separate dressing room, but Jarrett had an opportunity to pop his head into each room and meet the guests, basically just long enough to say hello.

"The longest visit I had was with Lassie," Jarrett later recalled, with laughter. "The dog plopped its head down in my lap, and I couldn't get up for a few minutes. I guess you could say we bonded."

He did not meet Rosie beforehand. He was told she likes the audience to see natural first meetings.

A few minutes before ten, mom and dad wished their son good luck and offered a last piece of advice.

"Just be yourself. It will be over before you know it," they told him. But deep down, they were a little worried about what might come out of his mouth. Everything he had done on television to this point had been edited.

An assistant escorted them to a couple of seats in the audience, where they held their breath and watched the clock, getting more nervous by the minute. Backstage, Jarrett petted Lassie.

Twenty-five minutes into the show, Rosie introduced Jarrett.

"My next guest is truly inspirational. He turns rainy days into sunny ones for every child he meets. He has a heart of gold and on top of that, he's only ten years old. Please welcome Jarrett Mynear!"

The band struck up the theme music, and the camera panned to the left of the stage. Jarrett, dressed in a plaid short-sleeved shirt, limped down two steps and waved to the crowd, which applauded loudly. He carried something in his left hand, but it wasn't clear what it was. He walked to center stage where Rosie stood to meet him and shook her hand.

Jennifer and Doug sat on the edge of their seats, beaming on the outside, tied in knots on the inside.

Rosie told Jarrett she had seen the news story about him and was impressed.

"Tell everyone what you do."

"Well," began Jarrett, "I have a business that I started. I take around three carts of toys to the kids at the Children's Hospital in Kentucky."

He looked straight into the camera as he continued, like an old pro who wants to make sure the audience is included in the conversation.

"Each kid gets to pick a toy of their choice. They're brand new and so far, we've had a great response, and everybody thinks it's a good idea."

If he was nervous, it didn't show.

Rosie asked Jarrett how he got the idea for the cart. He told her about his time in the Seattle hospital and how the ladies auxiliary there brought toys around.

"It always helped me look forward to something, and I wasn't quite as scared when I knew that they were coming around," he said. "I thought maybe I could do something like that to help the kids who are really scared and some of the kids who are new at this and some of the ones who are old at this."

Rosie asked him why he had been in the hospital so often. Jarrett calmly and clearly explained his three bouts with Ewing's sarcoma, once in the leg and twice in the lining of his skull.

"Then I had myelodysplasia, which is a bone marrow cancer and it can turn into leukemia, but they got it before it did."

The audience erupted into applause with that last piece of good news. Jarrett responded with a giant smile.

Then, Rosie had her director roll some of our videotape so the audience could see Jarrett in action, taking toys from room to room at the UK Children's Hospital.

"Were the kids surprised when you first showed up with the toys?" the host asked.

"Yes," answered Jarrett. "One of the fathers of one of the kids tried to pull out his wallet and was wondering how much the toy cost. I said it was free. You don't have to pay for anything on the cart."

"Well, Jarrett, that brings up a good point. How do you get all these brand new toys?"

"I have some private donors who give money and donate some toys, too," he said. "I've contacted businesses and stores that have been really nice to donate toys."

"Where do you keep all the toys?"

"In our family room."

"In your family room?!" Rosie asked, wide-eyed and incredulously.

"That's right," Jarrett laughed. Then he turned and looked straight into the camera again. His voice raised an octave and several decibels as he spread out his hands for emphasis.

"And if anybody can, WE NEED SOMEONE TO DONATE A WAREHOUSE!"

The audience broke out in loud laughter.

"Guess what, Jarrett?" Rosie exclaimed. "You now have a warehouse, and Toys "R" Us is going to stock it with as many toys as you need."

Jarrett's eyes got big and his smile even bigger. He seemed speechless, but the audience could read his lips as he mouthed, "Oh, my gosh."

"You keep doing what you do," Rosie ordered. "I think it's a great thing."

Then she prompted him to talk about the little girl who hadn't gotten out of bed for days—the same story he had told me during our interview.

"She got up and got something off the cart and ran back to bed and started playing with it. I just thought that was so nice. I'm glad I can make that much of a difference in these kids' lives."

He said it humbly, not boastfully.

"We're glad you can too, Jarrett," said Rosie. "Very glad."

Then she touched on another subject dear to Jarrett's heart. She held up a picture of his cabin mates from Indian Summer Camp, relating how they had whisked Jarrett away from one of his favorite places on a day's notice.

"That must be a special camp you go to," she said.

"Yes, it's a camp for cancer kids. And this is my cabin. Cabin Number Eleven!" Jarrett announced with enthusiasm.

Everyone applauded for Cabin Number Eleven. Jarrett knew his buddies would be watching with pride back in Kentucky.

Then Rosie mentioned that she had heard Jarrett had tried to go to FAO Schwarz.

"Yes," he said. "I was going to get all this *Star Wars* stuff and they were closed for a special meeting."

"They were closed!" Rosie seemed indignant. "Were you going to get it for you or the kids at the hospital or both?"

"Both," Jarrett laughed sheepishly. "I'm looking for this Lego set and I can't find it in Kentucky."

Rosie instructed Jarrett to say "abracadabra."

"Abracadabra," Jarrett obeyed, watching as Rosie reached beneath her desk.

She pulled out a *Star Wars* Lego set and handed it to the boy.

"Whoaaa!" Jarrett exclaimed, again turning temporarily speechless.

In the audience, Doug and Jennifer marveled at how the staffers had picked up on everything they had heard in the dressing room and made magic happen in such a short span of time.

"I guess you have to watch what you say around here," Jennifer whispered to her husband.

Back on stage, it was obvious Rosie was about to wrap up the interview. It had gone six minutes, which is about standard for a segment on a television talk show.

"I have a gift for you, too," Jarrett told Rosie.

"What do you have for me?"

He reached beside his seat and held up that item he had carried out from backstage.

"At Indian Summer Camp this year, there was a special gift for each kid. This is a flashlight and when you pull on it, it turns into a lantern," he said as he demonstrated.

"I signed it for you."

Again, the audience roared its approval.

"I thank you very much, mister. Give me a high five."

Jarrett slapped Rosie's hand.

"I'll treasure it always," she said. "It was nice to meet you, honey. Keep up the good work."

"Great meeting you," Jarrett said.

And the show went to a commercial break.

Doug and Jennifer got up from their seats to go meet their son backstage.

They knew he had just been given a dose of medicine that was better than anything in a bottle.

It was like a booster shot of spirit.

After the show, Rosie came back out on stage to pose for pictures with the guests and audience members and to sign autographs.

Doug and Jennifer met her.

"She was wonderful," Jennifer said. "She talked to us like we had known her for years. In fact, everyone from the show came back out and just made over Jarrett, telling him what a good job he did. It was obvious they were smitten with him."

Rosie pulled Jennifer aside.

"I want to know how he's really doing," Rosie said.

Jennifer told her that Jarrett's situation was always a "one day at a time" thing.

"But right now, things really are looking up."

"I'll keep in touch," Rosie said. And in the months to come, she was true to that promise.

The family made another friend that day, someone who, like Rosie, continued to call and check on Jarrett's progress long after the taping was a distant memory. Joey Kola was the show's audience coach, the one who comes out before the show and tells jokes, encourages applause, and goes over the rules of being in a studio audience.

He came up to Jarrett afterward, with tears in his eyes.

"I'm as sincere as I've ever been," he told the ten-year-old. "I've met a lot of stars on this show and big name athletes, but it means more to me to meet you than all of them put together. People say those people are heroes. To me, you're what's really a hero."

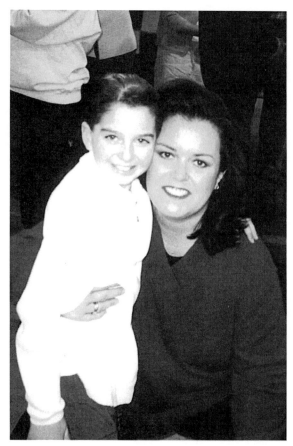

Jarrett and Rosie O'Donnell, June 1999

27

Toyland

As the Mynears gathered their things to leave the NBC studios, a production assistant came up to them and asked them how much time they had before they had to be at the airport.

Doug checked his watch and said they had about ninety minutes to kill.

"Good," the assistant said. "How would you like to go to FAO Schwarz?"

As had happened so often that morning, a big smile crossed Jarrett's face. Someone at the world's largest toy store had just seen the live broadcast of *The Rosie O'Donnell Show* and called to offer the Mynears a private tour. The CEO wanted Jarrett to be his guest. He had been impressed by the young man and dismayed that he had been unable to visit the night before.

Even Rosie's staff, which was used to pulling off all kind of surprises, was caught off guard by the call.

A limo was already waiting out front.

So off they went. In a matter of minutes, the car pulled up in front of the store and a man dressed like a giant toy soldier opened the limo door and escorted the family to the store's entrance.

"There were a lot of tourists standing around on the plaza," Jennifer laughed. "No doubt, they were wondering what celebrity had just arrived. Maybe they thought it was going to be Michael Jackson or McCauley Caulkin. Then we got out. They had to wonder who in the world we were."

Surprisingly, a couple of people knew.

Doug overheard one woman say, "I just saw that boy on the Rosie show." And another woman approached the Mynears to let them know she was from Louisville. She had seen stories about Jarrett back home in Kentucky.

That's the power of television. Instant recognition. It was an Andy Warhol moment, although Jarrett's fame was going to last a lot more than fifteen minutes.

"I thought to myself what a whirlwind we were in," Jennifer said. "On Monday, I had been washing floors at home. I got a phone call from New York, and now it was forty-eight hours later and we were in the spotlight. It was surreal."

Inside, the store's CEO, several managers, and the marketing director greeted the family and told Jarrett how honored they were that he wanted to visit their store. Then they whisked him straight to the *Star Wars* room. The first thing Jarrett noticed was the Darth Maul costume.

His mom described his reaction as "bug-eyed."

Every piece of *Star Wars* merchandise ever produced must have been in that room.

As Jarrett studied the displays, both the manager and an assistant manager came up with baskets in their hands.

"Let's pick some things out," they told Jarrett. "Get anything you want."

"Thanks so much," Jarrett said. "Some of this stuff will be so cool to have on The Joy Cart."

"No, we mean pick some things out for yourself," the manager said. "We're going to take care of The Joy Cart, too, but right now we want to treat you."

As they walked the aisles, the managers kept pointing to things, asking Jarrett if he would like to have this or that.

"It's funny," his mother said. "They almost had to make him take things. He was just overwhelmed. He really must have thought he didn't deserve all the attention. I would have guessed that he would have taken everything he could get his hands on. But he wasn't greedy at all. The people in the store really wanted to pile on the gifts."

As they walked through the various rooms, one of the employees learned that Jarrett had a sister back home. So, they took him to the Madeline room so he could pick out a doll for Claire.

Then Jarrett noticed a large stuffed frog.

"My granny would love that."

The manager asked why he thought so.

Jarrett told them that Granny Jeanne had given him several small frogs over the years, ever since she had accidentally killed one in her bedroom. She told him to sit them on the dressers in his hospital rooms. When he looked at the frogs, she wanted him to think of her and know that she was always thinking of him.

"Well, let's wrap it up for her," the manager said.

"Jarrett," his mother interrupted. "We'll never be able to get that big thing back on the plane."

She was told not to worry about that. The store would ship everything out that evening. It would arrive in Kentucky by courier the next day.

Time was running out, but the folks in the store had one more place to show Jarrett. It was a private room that was more like a museum of the world's most exclusive and expensive toys. It was a place for celebrities, not open to the public.

The room contained a toy Mercedes Benz and $25,000 dolls bedecked with jewels. Each corner contained virtual reality games and some of the most elaborate pinball machines ever built. A massive model train display took up a large portion of floor space. Everything was turned on and Jarrett was allowed to play with anything he wanted.

It was the stuff fairy tales are made of—"The Frog and the Little Prince: Chapter One—The Secret Chamber."

Jarrett had been in a hurry to get back to camp, but that was before he discovered the hidden rooms of FAO Schwarz. He could've stayed there well into the night.

On the way out of the store, the Mynears passed through the candy department. One of the assistants asked Jennifer how many kids were at Jarrett's camp.

When she found out it was about eighty, she didn't blink an eye.

"Let's send something back for them," the assistant said.

She suggested a new type of lollipop that used batteries in the handle. When you placed the candy in your mouth, you could hear songs play in your head.

Jarrett sampled one and thought it was pretty cool. So, they bagged up eighty of them and handed them to Jarrett. Once again, he was going to get to play Santa Claus.

By late afternoon, the Mynears pulled into Indian Summer Camp. Jarrett— in fact, everyone—was exhausted. But it was a hero's welcome.

One of the meeting rooms had been turned into a party room. All of the campers came in for ice cream, and they watched a tape of Jarrett's appearance with Rosie. Jarrett grinned from ear to ear as he saw his interview played back for the first time. Everyone cheered when he mentioned the camp.

Then he passed out the suckers, and eighty kids spent the next hour listening to voices in their heads.

Night fell, and everyone made their way back to their cabins, using their special camp flashlights.

As he approached Cabin Number Eleven, Jarrett wondered if Rosie was using the one he had given her.

28

Response

The talk show appearance opened the floodgates of goodwill. Jarrett's family began to receive donations and letters from across the country.

"Vacation Bible Schools from all over Kentucky told us they wanted to make The Joy Cart their fundraising project," Jennifer said. "We would get checks for $1,000 or $1,500. The teachers would attach letters saying they had never collected that much before."

The toy cart was something to which kids everywhere could relate. They could really see how their money was being put to good use, and a lot of them emptied their piggy banks to help.

Guy Jones, a children's minister at Burlington First Church of Christ in northern Kentucky, knew as soon as he heard about Jarrett's Joy Cart that it would spark generosity in young people. His church began an annual "Christmas in July" event to benefit The Joy Cart.

He transformed the church parking lot into a water park, with sprinklers, slides, and water balloons. A Christmas tree was the centerpiece, and Santa appeared wearing a Hawaiian shirt and swim trunks. Children put hundreds of toys under the tree for the cart.

"Once you started helping, you couldn't stop," Guy said.

Jarrett's Joy Cart also became the pet project for countless civic groups. Just as Rosie O'Donnell had promised, a warehouse became available in Lexington, donated by Rob McGoodwin of McGoodwin Records Management. The Mynears hauled several pickup loads of toys out of their basement family room to the new wide-open space. And within a couple of weeks, a tractor trailer pulled up to the warehouse, loaded with games, action figures, dolls, and stuffed animals from Toys "R" Us.

"Looking at it, it was hard to imagine that I had worried so that we wouldn't be able to keep the toy cart going after a couple of trips," Jennifer said. "It was overwhelming."

Not only did they have enough toys to give out fifty each week at the UK Children's Hospital, they had extras to give to charity auctions, to families who had been burned out of their homes, to a shelter for abused children and runaways, and to Christmas toy drives. They also put smaller items in the oncology clinic's "treasure chest." Then, when kids came in for blood tests, infusions, and other procedures, they could take home stickers, beanie babies, or bouncy balls as a reward for being brave.

Each year, the American Cancer Society sponsors hundreds of fundraisers around the country. Relay for Life is the biggest one in communities from coast to coast. Participants solicit donations and walk for miles, often around a high school track.

At the 1999 relay in Lexington, Jarrett was the star. His friend Kathy Tabb had asked him to read the ACS mission statement before the walkers took off around the track at Henry Clay High School.

Jarrett stood at the microphone and read how the organization works to "offer hope, progress and answers" to those who battle the world's most widespread disease.

"Here was this little person standing there not ashamed that he didn't have hair, not self-conscious of his size or hung up in any way about his condition," Kathy said. "Just the few words he had to say made more of an impact than anything anyone else could have done. I had more than a few adults say Jarrett has changed the entire way they look at having cancer."

After his opening remarks, Jarrett grabbed a corner of a banner that said "Cancer Survivors Thank You for Your Support" and led the walkers around the track, moving alongside Norma Akers, one of his favorite nurses. She was a breast cancer survivor. He had on sunglasses, his cap was turned backward, and he had on shorts—not embarrassed at all that his prosthesis was showing.

Except for the artificial leg, he looked just like any other cool kid hanging out behind the school.

"After that, I couldn't believe how many people sought him out just to shake his hand or get his autograph," Kathy said. "They were gushing over him as if he were the biggest movie star or athlete in the world. He was giving pep talks left and right."

She realized then that her young friend's giving wasn't just in the form of toys. The way he inspired people was greater than any gift one could hold in their hands.

That fall, Jarrett's classmates at West Jessamine Middle School sponsored their first major toy drive. They set up a Giving Tree in the school's lobby, and students were encouraged to take a tag from its branches. The tags were generic enough, saying things as simple as "Buy a gift appropriate for a five-year-old girl" or "Buy a book that would interest a ten-year-old boy."

Most kids went above and beyond what the tags said. If they were asked to buy a book, many of them bought ten books instead.

"That's what was so dumbfounding to us," Jennifer said. "We didn't know how it would mushroom and affect everyone in the school. The generosity was infectious. Jarrett may have looked different than the other kids and he was about half their size, but they saw how he was reaching out and wanted to be a part of it."

Many of the school's clubs, such as the Future Community Career Leaders of America, got involved in the drive. Long after the last tag was taken off the tree, students were still collecting toys.

"I've never seen anything bring a school together like that," said Jennifer, who had been a teacher for years. "When I would walk into the school with Jarrett, it never ceased to amaze me the reaction he would get. Everyone stopped to talk to him."

Every school has its cliques, close-knit groups of students who are considered to be bookworms and nerds, and those who are jocks and the "popular people." Jarrett seemed to fit into any group. He was never shunned and seldom teased among his peers.

Students yelled their greetings from the other end of hallways, gave him high fives, and offered to open doors or carry his books any time they could.

"I came close to crying so many times just by walking down the hall," Jarrett's mother said. "Everyone made sure Jarrett fit in. The principal once introduced him at an assembly as someone who was small in stature but huge in heart. Those words really made Jarrett feel good."

Jarrett and his mother were asked to visit the students in the Alternative School, a separate area for those who had difficulty adjusting to the structure of a classroom. Many of the kids were from broken homes and had already been in trouble with the law. They were prone to fights, destined to drop out, and generally didn't care that much about homework or class rank.

"But when we went in there, the kids could not have been sweeter," Jennifer said. "They showed us great respect. They called me Mrs. Mynear and offered me their chairs. They all shook Jarrett's hand, and many of them said they would be bringing toys in to help. Their teachers said they had never seen those kids pay so much attention to a guest."

There really was something magical about Jarrett. He tore down walls, made mean people nice, tough people cry, and sad people smile.

When the toy drive ended, the gifts were stacked taller than the tree and pretty much took over the lobby. It was the definition of school pride, embodied in boxes and bags.

As the collection effort wound down, Jarrett's family received another stack of papers to fill out. But these documents didn't outline the risks of experimental surgeries, have anything to do with insurance or drug plans, or contain medical terms and procedures with definitions too complicated to comprehend.

They were nomination forms for a major national award. Kathy Tabb, who later became president of the local chapter of the American Cancer Society, presented it to the Mynears. It was a big surprise. Kathy had secretly worked to push Jarrett's name for the Prudential Spirit of Community Awards.

One hundred and four students would be chosen nationwide to compete for ten national medals. The finalists would include two students from each state, the District of Columbia, and Puerto Rico. Half of them would be middle schoolers and the other half would come from the high school level.

The Prudential Insurance Company received more than twenty thousand applications.

"We were glad to fill out the forms—mostly as a favor to Kathy—but we didn't really think too much about winning," Jennifer said. "The odds against it were incredible, and there were so many worthy applicants."

But the word came in February that Jarrett would be Kentucky's middle school winner. Prudential wanted to make the presentation in front of the student body at Jarrett's school.

The principal called an assembly, but the students didn't really know what was up.

A representative of the insurance company took the microphone and began to talk about the award and what community spirit meant. The kids caught on pretty quickly. They began to whisper that "it must be for Jarrett." They spied Jarrett's parents in the back of the room.

After a few minutes, their suspicions were confirmed. When Jarrett was called to the podium, students and teachers jumped to their feet, cheering and applauding loudly. A large silver medallion was placed over Jarrett's head.

It was seen as an award for the whole school and, in part, it was. The response to the toy drive had been one of the factors that had made an impression on the judges.

"I have something else for Jarrett," the presenter continued. "Here's a check for $1,000."

More applause and open-mouthed expressions resulted. That was an awfully big number to put on a check. To the students, it might as well have been a million dollars.

"And Jarrett gets an all-expenses paid trip to Washington, D.C. This May, he'll represent Jessamine County and Kentucky in the national competition."

Jarrett was on cloud nine as his classmates patted him on the back and asked to see the medal.

He wasn't sure he could win at a higher level. His classmates didn't see how he could lose.

29

Common Bond

Jarrett's circle of friends included a lot of kids with cancer. When he wheeled The Joy Cart into a room at the UK Children's Hospital, Jarrett's first question to a new patient was almost always "What are you in here for?"

He would compare notes with the children, asking them which doctors they knew, how long they would be receiving chemotherapy, and so on.

"Well, hang in there. It's not so bad," he would say. "I've been through it four times."

You could see apprehension vanish as Jarrett talked to the patients, completely tuning out the other adults in the room. Many scared kids realized if this little guy could handle it, so could they.

Jarrett actually began those goodwill visits around the hospital months before he began thinking about The Joy Cart.

In 1997, Jarrett met Charles Ballard Wolford, a boy who was five years older than he, from the small eastern Kentucky town of Phelps. Everyone called him C. B.

C. B. also had Ewing's sarcoma. A few weeks after he began his chemotherapy, his weight dropped from ninety pounds to fifty-nine pounds. He had violent reactions to the treatment, throwing up several times a day. According to his mother, Faye Wolford, C. B. completely lost his will to live.

"He was really depressed," Faye said. "He wouldn't talk. He wouldn't do anything. He said he wanted to die."

Enter Jarrett.

The pint-sized cheerleader learned that C. B. had given up hope. So, he made a visit to his room.

"He pops in the door and says, 'Hey man, you're not dead yet. Let's have some fun,'" Faye said. "He wanted C. B. to play Nintendo with him."

But C. B. said he didn't feel like it.

"Yeah, yeah, come on," Jarrett insisted. "I need somebody to beat."

Faye recalled an instant change in C. B.'s demeanor.

"C. B. was sitting there looking at this little guy who's been through everything he's been through . . . same cancer . . . and he came out of that bed and started playing video games. From that moment on, this kid did not stop."

She watched the two boys as they laughed and played for more than an hour.

"It was like a miracle. It was wonderful," she said. "Jarrett gave me my boy back."

Jarrett and C. B. had many discussions about what to anticipate with the bone marrow transplant and how he could expect to feel after taking different medicines.

The two became close pals, not only around the hospital, but also at summer camp.

As C. B.'s condition worsened, he decided to write a book. That effort gained him a lot of attention.

Through a chain of events that began with a pen pals program at the hospital, news of C. B's book made it to an aide at the White House. On a chilly October morning in 1998, C. B. picked up the phone at his home and mumbled a few words into the receiver.

He called to his mother: "Mom, it's the White House. They want to speak to you."

Faye told him to quit kidding around.

"No really, Mom, I think it's for real," C. B. said.

Faye took the phone and listened as a liaison for President Bill Clinton invited the family to come to Washington for a visit.

Faye began to cry. C. B. had dreamed of meeting the President, but she never believed it would be possible.

Friends and family members, as well as people from the hospital (including the Mynears), pitched in to help pay for a trip to the nation's capital. On October 11th, C. B. toured the White House and sat in on the President's weekly radio address to the nation. After the broadcast, Mr. Clinton came over and introduced himself to C. B. They posed for pictures, and C. B. got to sit in the President's chair. According to his mother, the young man was extremely sick that day, but he put on a brave face, telling the President he was doing well.

Just sixteen days later, C. B. died.

In the months that followed, his mother finished his book.

That spring, as the school day ended at West Jessamine Middle School, Jarrett went to the car where his mother was waiting for him.

She held a book.

"I want you to look at this," Jennifer said, handing the book to Jarrett.

It was *My Story About Cancer* by Charles B. Wolford (Seven Locks Press, 1999).

"Look inside," she instructed.

Jarrett opened the cover and read the dedication:

"To my best friend, Jarrett."

Response to Jarrett's first appearance on *The Rosie O'Donnell Show* had been so great that the producers decided to invite him back for an update in February 2000.

Jarrett said he would love to come back and he wanted to mention C. B.'s book.

So the producers also invited Faye Wolford to be a guest.

Doug and Jennifer enjoyed escorting Faye and her sister around The Big Apple. It was the first time C. B.'s mom and aunt had seen the skyscrapers of New York City, and it was a delight for the women from the coalfields of eastern Kentucky.

"We all laughed constantly," Jennifer said. "We looked like the typical tourists, with our necks craned upward and our jaws gaping open at the sights. Doug was determined to show them as much as he could in one night. He wore us all out the night before the show."

They went to the top of the Empire State Building, to Radio City Music Hall, and to the lobby of the World Trade Center. They were out until midnight.

It didn't matter. No one could sleep anyway.

During the warm-up before the live broadcast the next morning, one man in the audience seemed disappointed when he heard the topic would be "children who make a difference."

He yelled out that he wanted to see celebrities.

Jennifer said the audience coach, their friend Joey Kola, went off on the man.

"Let me tell you," Joey said emphatically, "these people you'll see today are more like stars than anyone you could ever meet!"

As the segment about Jarrett was introduced, a videotape played that gave the audience background about his relationship with C. B.

The tape included a home video clip with C. B. near the end of his life, with sunken cheeks and pale skin. He said, in a weak voice with a heavy Southern accent, "The way I feel is you fight until you can't fight no more."

Then Jarrett appeared on the tape, with tears streaming down his face, saying, "I just want everybody to know that he was a great boy and that he wanted to help everyone. I think that's great."

Jarrett and Faye received warm applause as the tape ended, and the cameras cut to them live on stage.

Faye told how C. B. had mentioned to her as soon as he started the book that he wanted to dedicate it to Jarrett.

"I asked him why," Faye said softly "And he said "Jarrett just inspires me.'"

Faye took Jarrett's hand, and Jarrett's smile reached from ear to ear. They both felt C.B's spirit was with them.

Then Rosie called attention to the silver medallion hanging around Jarrett's neck.

"What's that new necklace you're wearing? Are you stylin'?" she teased.

"No, I don't wear ten-ton weights just for style," Jarrett said, laughing.

"Good, good," said Rosie. "So what is it? Did you win the Olympics?"

Jarrett explained that he was a local winner of the Prudential Spirit of Community award and that he would soon be going to Washington to compete for a national honor.

Again, loud applause filled the studio.

"And what does that say about volunteering?" Rosie prompted.

Jarrett ended the show with great words of wisdom.

"I think anybody, no matter what age they are, can get into volunteering—that they can help somebody. That completes your life. It makes it worthwhile."

30

Metal Head

"Routine scans" became a dreaded term for the Mynears. Doctors used the phrase to mean there's nothing to worry about: "We're just checking to make sure everything's as good as we think it is."

But so many times the results had meant the *routine* would be months of chemo treatments and radiation. Each time Jarrett's parents took him in for an MRI, a CAT scan, or an x-ray, there was nervousness in the air. Too many times the films showed mysterious dark spots in bones and tissue.

On March 27, 2000, just three weeks from Jarrett's eleventh birthday, the *routine* played out again.

This time the scans showed cancer had returned in the lining of Jarrett's skull and was dangerously close to the brain.

Ewing's sarcoma was back for the fourth time.

"We were scared to death," Jarrett's mother recalled. "Now the doctors were talking about making incisions in the top of Jarrett's head—cuts that would be just centimeters from his brain."

They wondered if just a little slip of the hand could result in permanent brain damage. But, again, they were overcome with that inevitable feeling of blind faith. What other choice did they have?

"The doctors were careful to stress to us that this was in the *lining* of the skull and the *lining* of the brain, not in the brain itself," Jennifer said. The indication was that it would move into the brain if they did not act soon.

So, within a week, Jarrett was back on the operating table. The doctors made a slit down the back of his head and pulled the skin apart. They removed a piece of bone from his skull about four inches in diameter and scraped tumor tissue off the brain's lining.

The operation went on for a half day as the surgeons worked with care and precision. Jarrett's head was in a vice to keep him from moving even the slightest bit while he slept.

When they were certain they had removed as much of the cancerous tissue as possible, the doctors sized a piece of metal to put in Jarrett's head to replace the missing section of skull. That act meant a new nickname for the boy. In the weeks and months to come, Jennifer began calling Jarrett "Titanium Head" whenever they got into a good-natured teasing match.

Anyone who looked closely could see the screws under the skin on Jarrett's head and, in typical fashion, he made the most of his unique circumstances. Jarrett liked to shock people by telling them about the metal plate and showing them its outline.

He told airport security guards that he was "their walking nightmare." If the plate in his head didn't set off metal detectors, his prosthesis was sure to. He was the "bionic man." If he was going to set off bells and whistles at the airport, he might as well enjoy the attention. He left guards and everyone behind him laughing each time he finally got clearance to pass through the checkpoints.

He would walk through the metal detector with his hands straight in front of him and step without bending at the knees—just like Frankenstein's monster, groaning and glaring straight ahead. He had a knack for turning awkward moments into lighthearted encounters.

For several weeks, Jarrett received low levels of radiation beamed at his head.

"We worried about that, too," Jennifer said. "We were told that skin and bone could break down over time, but the doctors ended that treatment just as soon as they felt they could."

More chemotherapy followed, this time using Taxotere injections, a drug that was considered noninvasive and one that did not affect Jarrett's quality of life. It did not make him nauseous or zap his energy.

The chemo was to attack a part of the tumor that could not be removed during the surgery. According to Dr. Jeffrey Moscow, chief of pediatric hematology/oncology, that section of the tumor was attached to a large vein that drains part of the brain. The surgeons were concerned that entering that space would cause draining they could not control.

Jarrett rebounded quickly, shunning the helmet his radiologist wanted him to wear. Life's a journey, and Jarrett intended to stay on the road. He had a lot of appearances and trips coming up, and he wasn't about to miss them.

Jarrett was a man of steel, and he could tap on his head to prove it.

31

Medal Winner

In May, the Mynears went to Washington. It was still amazing to them that Jarrett's Joy Cart project had won them trips to New York and now, the nation's capital.

Along with the Prudential honor came four days of touring museums and historic sites, and several programs and seminars on volunteerism.

As the Mynears checked into the Marriott hotel in McLean, Virginia, headquarters for the ceremonies, they were separated from their son.

"We found out right away that for the next four days, the kids would stay together and the parents would stay together, but the two groups would have little contact," Jennifer said. "Jarrett was matched up with a roommate from another part of the country. Our rooms wouldn't even be on the same floor."

She praised the arrangement, saying it really helped the children hone their social skills.

"It was a fantastic experience. The kids made friends instantly," she said. "I'd never seen Jarrett so emotionally charged in his life."

On the first night, the students went through several ice-breaking exercises. They played games and then told about their own projects, the ones that had won them the honor to be there.

Jarrett cherished the interaction.

"My friends at school could talk about the toy cart, but they couldn't really relate to my reasons for doing what I do," Jarrett said. "But these kids were like me. It was so easy to talk to them about anything."

The group was described as the brains behind one hundred and four amazing ideas.

There were kids who started food kitchens in their neighborhoods, a boy who tested the quality of residential well water in his community, and those who devised anti-bullying programs in their schools and provided tutoring for slow learners. After reading about foster children who always seemed to be on the move and had to tote their belongings in plastic garbage bags, one girl collected suitcases for them. And there was Ryan Tripp, the famous "Lawnmower Boy" from Utah, who drew attention to the need for organ donors by mowing the lawns of capitol buildings in all fifty states.

One high school senior from Redmond, Washington, instantly became Jarrett's buddy. Paul Gordon had raised thousands of dollars for transplant patients and had become a national spokesman for the importance of organ donation. A year later, he would produce a documentary about young role models that included a profile of Jarrett.

"Everybody was pumped to be there," Jarrett said.

The week included a boat cruise on the Potomac River, a breakfast at the Capitol with U.S. senators and representatives, and a wreath-laying ceremony at the Tomb of the Unknown Soldier in Arlington National Cemetery.

On the second night, Senator John Glenn spoke to the group during a reception in the rotunda of the Museum of Natural History. Jarrett loved it. It was surreal to hear from one of the nation's space pioneers as he stood in the shadow of a giant wooly mammoth. The prehistoric past combined with 20th century history as an astronaut spoke about his accomplishments to those who would be leaders in the 21st century.

After the speech, many of the students went into a side room to have their pictures taken with the senator. As he waited his turn, Jarrett made another friend on the spot. His parents were shocked to see him walk out of the room holding the hand of a high-profile woman.

"Mom, Dad," Jarrett said. "This is Annie Glenn. She wanted to meet you."

And so they met the senator's wife. Doug and Jennifer never knew with whom their son was going to strike up a conversation.

Each day the nominees loaded onto buses to visit monuments and landmarks. The parents did the same thing, but on different buses with different destinations.

"It was amusing to see the adults heading in one direction and the kids going the other way," Jennifer said. "We would wave and acknowledge each other, and then wouldn't see each other again for hours."

It gave Jarrett a sense of freedom and responsibility.

The parents had no worries. Principals and school administrators from all over the country were there to serve as chaperones.

On the third day, all of the families gathered at the Reagan Building for the awards luncheon.

"Parents kept coming up to me and saying, 'You know Jarrett is going to be one of the winners, don't you?'" Jennifer said. "I didn't feel that way. All of the kids were winners, and I didn't see that he stood above any of them."

When Jarrett walked into the banquet hall, Jennifer gasped. She hadn't even been able to go to his room that morning to help him get ready for the ceremony.

There he stood, looking nice in his black suit and tie, but his shirttail wasn't completely tucked in and he had on blue sneakers. A baseball cap topped off the ensemble.

She looked at Doug and rolled her eyes. He laughed and said, "That's our boy!"

When the emcee announced the ten winners, sure enough Jarrett's name was called.

"It was mind-boggling," Jennifer said. "When I looked around that room and thought about all the things those one hundred and four kids had accomplished, I was so proud, not only of Jarrett but of America's youth. It was uplifting and reassuring. All of the kids were cheering. They celebrated each other."

In just three days, Jarrett had become close with three of the other four middle school winners. That made the celebration even more exciting.

There he stood on stage, now with a gold medallion around his neck and a baseball cap pulled down so far you couldn't see his eyes. But you could see the smile. It went from ear to ear.

The award included a $5,000 check to be used toward Jarrett's education. He also received a crystal bowl, etched with a drawing all around the rim of children holding hands.

When the ceremony ended, the other nominees were bused back to the hotel. But the winners stayed behind for pictures and radio interviews and to give quotes to be dropped into press releases. Once again, Jarrett wowed the reporters with his eloquence. In fact, his parents had trouble pulling him away. He wanted to talk to anyone and everyone who would listen.

"If I can do something like this, anyone can," he told the interviewers. "Volunteering just makes me feel so good."

You can bet that quote got used over and over by the public relations folks at Prudential.

"He was electrified," Jennifer said. "There's no doubt about it. I wouldn't take anything for that experience for him."

There was still another day of activities after the awards were handed out, and it held another lesson for Jarrett.

"I thought some of the kids might be jealous or down in the dumps about not winning," he said. "But the ones who didn't win were still nice. It was kind of weird. There was no jealousy."

Jarrett saw what it was like to be gracious in defeat. But really, it was a reflection of how he had been all his life. Each time he had been given disappointing news, he had refused to be down about it. He had always looked for things to celebrate.

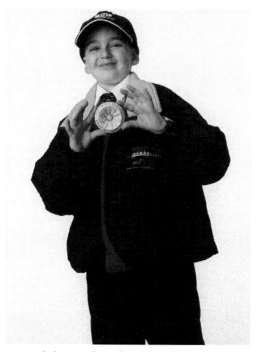

Jarrett with his Prudential Spirit of Community medal

32

Chance Meetings

Jarrett left Washington, knowing he would be back in just one month. He had learned earlier that year that he was a local recipient of a Jefferson Award.

The American Institute for Public Service each year recognizes people who encourage community involvement. The program has been around since 1962, when Jacqueline Kennedy Onassis, Senator Robert Taft, Jr., and philanthropist Sam Beard founded it. On the local level, media sponsors nominate ordinary people who do extraordinary things. WKYT-TV, the CBS affiliate in Lexington, nominated Jarrett. News Director Jim Ogle wrote that "Jarrett can inspire a room full of people more than any adult I've ever heard." Jarrett was one of forty-one local winners from more than fourteen thousand nominees nationwide.

There are also national winners—celebrities and politicians who have a long history of fostering public service. Past winners had included former Secretary of State Dr. Henry Kissinger, tennis great Arthur Ashe, and Supreme Court Justice Thurgood Marshall. The 2000 winners included country singer Faith Hill, who had established an adult literacy program, and Dr. Benjamin Carson, a world-renowned pediatric surgeon at John Hopkins University Hospital. Another familiar name appeared on the winner's list. U.S. Senator John Glenn would be recognized for his public service. So Jarrett was in elite company.

This trip allowed for winners to bring just one guest, so Doug stayed behind. Most of the winners were adults who brought spouses.

From the time they checked into the Loews L'Enfant Plaza Hotel and were ushered to the opening night cocktail reception, Jarrett and his mother could tell this was a highly formal and prestigious affair. It was a completely different atmosphere than the Prudential ceremony a month earlier where kids roamed the halls in t-shirts and shorts.

Jarrett felt a little uncomfortable at first, but at the reception each winner was asked to give a one-minute speech about his or her project. Again, he was impressed by all the good ideas these people had. There were people who established food banks, those who opened clinics in poor inner city neighborhoods, and athletes who spent countless hours in anti-drug outreach programs.

"They were adults who had the same motivations as he did," his mother said. "Before, he had mostly been exposed to kids who were working on projects through their schools or on their summer breaks."

Jarrett, who made friends quickly everywhere he went, did it again that first night at the hotel. After the reception, he struck up a conversation with another of the local award winners, Greg Forbes Siegman, a substitute teacher from Chicago. The twenty-seven-year-old had been mentioned in more than two hundred media reports and was one of the country's most celebrated volunteers.

Greg's story began in 1997 when he ran into two of his African-American students who lived in the Chicago projects and invited them into a restaurant to join him for milkshakes. The restaurant catered to mostly affluent white customers. When Greg and the students sat down, he noticed a woman at the next table look at them in disdain and move her purse out of reach. It made Greg furious, and he vowed to turn the negative into a positive. Since then, he had never missed a week of bringing different kids together for milkshakes and conversation. His "BrunchBunch.com" program included hundreds of students and adults from different races, cultures, and financial backgrounds. The lunches took place in more than fifty of Chicago's nicest restaurants, and from that effort Greg was able to form a foundation that gives scholarships to young people who could have never dreamed of going to college. He called it the 11-10-02 Foundation, naming it for his yet-to-come thirtieth birthday. Greg wanted the name to symbolize how much can be accomplished by people in their younger years.

During a group photo session following the reception, Greg was asked to kneel down on the floor with the four teen winners while the adult winners stood behind them.

"I was insulted," Greg said, not seriously. "I had gone there determined to act like an adult, even though I was the youngest of the adult winners. And here was the photographer lumping me in with the kids. But it turned out to be a blessing because that's how I met Jarrett."

"Greg and Jarrett just hit it off," Jennifer said. "Jarrett loved hearing Greg's stories and, even though he had done such important things, Greg was just like a big kid. His enthusiasm was contagious."

Greg had shaved his head just before his trip to Washington because he had lost a Super Bowl bet. Jennifer noted that Jarrett looked like Greg's "Mini-Me."

After the two talked for about a half-hour, Jarrett excused himself to go to the restroom. Greg, who obviously was accustomed to doing things on a whim, asked Jennifer if she thought Jarrett would like to go on a tour of the White House.

"I said *we'd* love to go," Jennifer said.

Greg had a high school friend who worked in the mailroom at the White House, and she had arranged for him to visit the next afternoon. He said he would make a call to see if he could bring another guest.

The next morning, the Mynears went to the National Press Club to listen to a panel discussion entitled "The 2000 Elections: Will America Vote?"

Corbin Bernsen, an actor best known for his years on the television drama *L.A. Law*, emceed. A camera crew taped the event, which was to be part of a television special about the Jefferson Awards. Bernsen would also narrate that.

To Jarrett, the discussion seemed to go on forever. The attention span of an eleven-year-old boy is only so long. The speakers fascinated Jennifer, but she could tell Jarrett was restless.

As the discussion wound down, Bernsen opened the floor to comments. He wanted to know if those who volunteer for community service are more likely to vote than other Americans. And he asked what could be done to get more young people involved in the political process. Jennifer gasped as she saw her son stand up. He stepped into the aisle and took a microphone.

"Adults need to realize they can't do everything on their own," Jarrett said. "There are a lot of kids who could really help out with community projects if they were just asked. My friends have never said 'no' when someone asked them to help. But they have to be asked.

"If they start seeing that they can make a difference when they're young, then I think they'll realize they can make a difference by voting when they're old enough. Kids are caught up in what's cool and what's not cool. America needs to make it cool to be someone who does community service."

Bernsen asked Jarrett for his name and told him he made a really good point.

"Thanks, Jarrett, for helping us look at this from a young person's point of view," the actor said.

Jennifer breathed a sigh of relief, wondering again where her son got all his courage.

After lunch, Jarrett and Jennifer went to the hotel lobby, geared up for a visit to the White House. Greg and his friend Shani Mott, his guest for the Jefferson Awards ceremonies, were already there, ready to go. Unfortunately, the Secret Service couldn't grant security clearance for Jennifer to go on such short notice. But Jarrett was allowed to be added to the guest list.

"I guess there's not much background to check on an eleven-year-old boy," Jennifer laughed. "I, however, could've had a long history of problems."

So, the trio headed down Pennsylvania Avenue on foot, promising to tell Jennifer all about it when they got back.

Jennifer decided to spend her time at the Natural History Museum. As she left the hotel, she questioned her judgment just for a moment.

"Here I was sending my son off with a guy I didn't even know, trusting his every word. But it seemed like such a great opportunity for Jarrett, I didn't want him to miss it."

The visit was just to be to the correspondence area, to see where students opened mail, stuffed envelopes, and basically worked as gophers for the White House staff.

As the quick visit neared an end, Jarrett had a parting thought.

"Could we meet the President's pets—Buddy the dog and Socks the cat?"

"Most people would never dream of asking such a thing," Greg said. "But Jarrett's mentality is to seize all opportunities. You never know what can happen if you don't ask."

To Greg's surprise, a White House aide told them she would try to arrange for Jarrett to see the animals. She told them to come back in a couple of hours, demonstrating how difficult it was to deny a sincere request from Jarrett.

Greg was as bold as his new friend.

"We'd like to meet the President, too," he said.

The woman smiled.

"That's not going to happen," she said.

"But," Greg protested, "I've been compared to Forrest Gump, and Forrest got to meet the President."

Back home in Chicago, Greg was known by many for his tendency to walk into unlikely circumstances, just like the movie character.

"You may meet his dog," the woman said. "That's as close as you're going to get."

Two hours later, Jarrett, Greg, and Shani started down Pennsylvania Avenue again for their second trip to the executive mansion. But they had to swing by a designated location to meet up with a fourth guest—Corbin Bernsen.

They had run into the actor on a D.C. sidewalk after the first White House visit and invited him to go, too. He had some free time and readily accepted.

"Apparently, they had no trouble getting *him* clearance," Jennifer said, feigning jealousy. "They must already have records on well-known people."

Off they went—the actor, the teacher, and the cancer patient—walking toward the home of the President of the United States.

As the group made its way to the White House, Jarrett overheard several women on the street giggling and whispering.

"That's Corbin Bernsen." Or "Isn't that the guy from *L.A. Law*?"

The actor walked on, pretending not to hear.

"We teased him about his fans," Jarrett said. "I told him the women were really looking at us."

When they got to their destination, the presidential dog walker was waiting for them, with Buddy and Socks at his side.

Bill Clinton's famous first dog sniffed the visitors, and Jarrett stooped to scratch his head. So did Greg. But as he knelt, he stepped on Buddy's tail. The chocolate Labrador retriever gave a quick yelp, and Greg jumped back, horrified at the faux pas. Jarrett snickered and told Greg to be careful.

"You're going to get us thrown out of here," he said.

Jarrett gave the cat a quick pat, too, but it was Buddy who really interested him.

The dog seemed agitated. An aide suggested that it may be a good idea to take Buddy for a walk to settle him down.

"Could we do it?" Jarrett asked, excitedly.

Again, Greg was taken aback by his new friend's boldness.

"Jarrett just never acted like he was asking anything unreasonable. Position or protocol didn't impress him. He was just a kid with a 'why not?' attitude. He wasn't deterred by his age or that he may have been physically tired because of his condition. He literally jumped at chances that came his way."

Over the months that followed, Greg got to know Jarrett better.

"Jarrett was a kid who put on a strong face when he was around people," Greg said. "He had a karma about him that said he could deal with anything. What kind of kid would ask to walk the President's dog? The same kind of kid who thinks he's going to live forever."

The trainer handed the boy the leash. Five people filed behind Jarrett and Buddy—Greg and his friend, two White House aides, and Corbin Bernsen.

They walked down a long hallway. Actually, the dog walked Jarrett.

The entourage strolled through several sections of the historic building. Jarrett and Company saw the rooms the public can see on tours, but they also got a more behind-the-scenes look.

They went into the press briefing room, which Jarrett noted looks a lot bigger on TV. He stood behind the same podium the President uses.

Then they went into a kitchen area, used exclusively for preparing floral arrangements.

The size of the room fascinated Jarrett, with its sinks and counters and a huge selection of vases, pots, and utensils that lined the walls. The White House florist showed him a freezer room full of fresh flowers and told him how the arrangements were changed every day.

"It seemed more like what you'd expect in a hotel," Jarrett said. "It was hard to believe all of this was for a house where just one family lived."

Then the group moved on through a maze of hallways, not really sure where the guides were taking them. An aide told them they had to steer clear of the Oval Office, but she did direct them through the West Wing.

As they rounded a corner, a Secret Service agent appeared.

"Step to the right side of the hall," he ordered.

The entourage stopped and backed against the wall.

A large set of double doors opened, and out walked President Clinton with the President of Argentina.

Jarrett's mouth fell open. So did Greg's.

Greg reached in his pocket to pull out his camera. The White House aide shook her head and mouthed "no pictures." Greg put his hands back to his side and shrugged his shoulders as if to say, "You can't blame me for trying."

The President stopped walking, looked at Jarrett, and smiled.

"That dog looks familiar," he said.

"It should," Jarrett replied loudly. "It's your dog!"

Everybody laughed, and Greg said, "We're taking good care of him, Mr. President." He was afraid Jarrett would tell the President he stepped on Buddy's tail.

"I just gave him a 'be quiet' look, and he got the hint," Greg said.

Clinton laughed, thanked Jarrett for giving his dog some exercise, shook his hand, and continued down the hall. Corbin smiled, remaining unnoticed in the background.

The two world leaders walked outside onto the West Wing's portico so dozens of photographers on the lawn could take pictures from a distance.

And thus ended Jarrett's brush with the most powerful politician in the world.

The White House aide rolled her eyes at Greg and said, "You really are Forrest Gump."

When the group came back to the hotel, Jennifer could tell immediately that Greg and Jarrett were especially excited.

"Guess what, Mom," Jarrett said. "We met the President!"

Jennifer looked at Greg, who shook his head in confirmation.

"I thought they were pulling my leg," Jennifer said, "just trying to make me jealous because I didn't get to go along."

They were running late and everyone had to immediately jump on a bus for the next Jefferson Awards event.

"Greg and Jarrett were telling everyone on the bus about running into Bill Clinton, so then I knew it was true," Jennifer said.

She asked Jarrett to tell her all about it.

"I got to walk Buddy," Jarrett said. "He's a really nice dog."

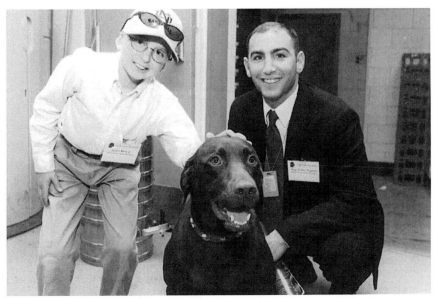

Jarrett and friend Greg Siegman in the West Wing of the White House with First Dog Buddy Clinton

33

Holding Court

After the White House experience, it was time to get back to business. Five local recipients of the Jefferson Award would receive yet another honor—the Jacqueline Kennedy Onassis Award for Greatest Public Service Benefiting Local Communities. They would be named at a banquet that night in the rotunda of the National Women in Arts Museum.

It was the fanciest dinner Jarrett had ever attended. All of the waiters wore tuxes. The rotunda was bathed in candlelight, and giant floral arrangements adorned each table. Each place setting contained the finest china and crystal wine glasses. Jarrett couldn't imagine why anyone needed that many forks, spoons, and knives.

There was one other small boy among the local winners—seven-year-old Trevor DeRuise, whose project was called "Lucky Ladybugs for Lupus." He had raised money for Lupus research by selling rocks painted to look like ladybugs. He and his mother were seated at the same table as Jarrett and Jennifer, along with a staffer from the Supreme Court and a board member of the Smithsonian Institution.

"Jarrett was starving," Jennifer said. "After all the running around at the White House, he didn't have time to get lunch. So he was really looking forward to the dinner."

But the menu wasn't designed for kids. The waiters stopped at their table with a large tray of meat lined with vegetables.

"I tried to pass it off as pork tenderloin and gravy, but I knew Jarrett wasn't going to like it," Jennifer said.

He took one bite and said he didn't like the texture.

"What is this, really?"

Jennifer told him it was duck.

The other boy at the table immediately began to shake. Images of Donald and Daffy ran through his head.

"I can't eat a duck," Trevor whispered.

"Me, either," said Jarrett.

"But Jarrett," Jennifer said, "you have to eat. You haven't had anything all day. It's not that bad."

In fact, she thought it was fantastic.

The others at the table also tried to convince the boys how good it was, but it was clear they weren't going to budge. To them, ducks were meant for feeding in ponds and laughing at in cartoons.

Trevor's mother whispered to Jennifer that there was a McDonald's across the street. She said she would slip out and get them Happy Meals. She said she would save them in her purse, and they could eat them later at the hotel. Jennifer nodded her approval.

"I did get Jarrett to eat the mashed potatoes," she said. "But as the night wore on, I could tell both boys were getting weak from hunger."

Finally, she decided there was no need to put on airs. She told the other mother just to go ahead and give the boys the Happy Meals right there at the table. There was no telling how late it would be when they got back to the hotel.

"It ended up being quite the topic of conversation," Jennifer laughed. "Many people came up to the table to talk to us, and all of them commented on the Happy Meals."

Many pictures were taken of the two boys sitting there in their suits, with tiny hamburgers laid out on fine china and cold fries spilled across a white tablecloth.

Jarrett was not named as one of the five national winners that night. He hadn't expected to be. But that did not mean his role in the event was finished.

Sam Beard, the co-founder and president of the American Institute for

Public Service, asked Jarrett to come to the final ceremony anyway. The five winners would be honored at the U.S. Supreme Court Building on the last morning. Mr. Beard wanted Jarrett to make a speech too, giving a child's perspective on what it means to be a volunteer. He had been impressed with the way Jarrett had handled interviews and the way he spoke up at the panel discussion.

That night, Jennifer tried to get Jarrett to write a speech in his hotel room. But he was tired.

"Don't worry, Mom," he told her. "I've been thinking about what to say. I have it inside my head."

That is exactly what worried her.

The next day, they showed up at the highest courthouse in the land. The ceremony took place in a conference area just off the main courtroom. A few minutes before it began, the Mynears were seated in the front row, facing a table of dignitaries. Jarrett immediately noticed Senator Glenn and waved at him. He was sure the former astronaut remembered him from his visit to D.C. a month earlier.

He must have because he made eye contact with his wife, who was standing along a side wall and nodded toward Jarrett. Annie Glenn came over and gave Jarrett a big hug and told him how good it was to see him again.

Then William Bennett, the nation's former Secretary of Education, came over to introduce himself. Next, a couple of well-known senators walked through the room. Jennifer told Jarrett who they were and then pointed out Justice Sandra Day O'Connor.

"I tried to tell Jarrett how important all these people in the room were," she said. "But he wasn't really fazed. He never thought of one person being any more important than another. To him, everyone was the same."

The ceremony was another one that ran longer than the organizers intended. It followed the formal rules of order where each presenter got multiple introductions. Jennifer thought they might nix Jarrett's speech in the interest of time.

But Sam Beard got up and nodded to Jarrett, indicating he would be next.

"This is when I usually make some closing remarks," Mr. Beard said. "But today, I want to give my time to someone very special whom I've asked to take my place. I'd like you to meet Jarrett Mynear."

Jarrett walked up to the podium, which bore the seal of the Supreme Court of the United States. His head could not be seen above it. Mr. Beard turned a chair around and lifted Jarrett up on it so he could speak into the microphone.

There was something very touching about the scene. Even before he spoke a word, Jennifer began to cry. She scanned the head table and noticed Corbin Bernsen was wiping away tears as well.

It was like years of memories were coming back to Jennifer at this one instant. She thought about all Jarrett had been through and had far he had come. So many times, she thought he would never live to see another day. Now, she could see clearly that God had a purpose for him. He had been allowed to live for a reason. He was a survivor who had gained an audience with some of the most influential people in the nation, and he had something to say they needed to hear. Sometimes, she thought, adults really do need a little child to lead them.

Because Jarrett wouldn't share his speech with her beforehand, she wondered if he was about to say something that would make her want to crawl under the table. Instead, she said it was the best speech he had ever given. It came from the heart, with no notes. He never stumbled or paused. The words just tumbled out of his mouth in an eloquence that seemed magical.

"Kids can do great things," Jarrett began. "They just need to be given support. People ask me why I started giving toys out to sick children in the hospital. It's because some adults did the same thing for me. I thought it was so nice that I wanted to do it, too. It made me feel better. It took my mind off my sickness. It kept me from feeling sorry for myself.

"Adults need to set a good example, and kids will take notice. Kids have good ideas, but adults have to make them happen. I couldn't have my Joy Cart if my parents didn't encourage me and help me get the donations and make the deliveries. A lot of adults got behind it and gave me money and toys. They never made me feel like it was a silly idea. They supported me.

"A lot of kids aren't as lucky as I am. They don't get that kind of support.

No one asks them what they think or seems to care.

"The media needs to get involved, too. They need to show the good things that kids are doing. We need to have more stories on the news that support kids and give them a chance. We hear a lot about the bad kids who take guns to school or do drugs, but we don't see that much about the ones who help collect toys or food or do nice things for people.

"We're the generation that's going to take over, but we need your help. Show us that there's nothing uncool about helping other people. Not everybody has to do something as big as my Joy Cart. But everybody can do something. Little things can make a big difference. I think that's the message we have to get out. It's not important what you do as long as you do something."

With that, Jarrett turned to Mr. Beard, indicating he was ready to be lifted from the chair. The audience members sat quiet for a moment, stunned at the impact of the short speech they had just heard. Again, Jennifer noticed a lot of teary eyes.

Then the applause came. And the little man who couldn't see over the podium seemed larger than life.

34
The Banquet and the Bishop

Among the many awards and trophies that line Jarrett's shelf at home, one of the most beautiful and meaningful is a crystal Madonna—the Queen of Heaven statuette.

Parishioners at the family's church, Mary Queen of the Holy Rosary, nominated Jarrett for the Bishop's Award, one of five honors to be given out at the annual Eastern Kentucky Diocesan Recognition Banquet in 2000.

It was no surprise to those who nominated him when the word came that Jarrett had won.

"This award really meant a lot to us," Jennifer said. "It said that Jarrett was being a Christian witness to others."

Jarrett was all smiles at the awards banquet, looking sharp in his suit and tie. This time, he made sure his shirt was tucked in and his shoes were shiny.

When he was able, Jarrett often served as an altar boy at church, and he had developed a special bond with a young associate pastor. Father Linh Nguyen, who had grown up in Vietnam, was described by many as "a big kid." He and Jarrett often got into verbal teasing matches.

At the banquet, in the main hall of a Lexington hotel, Jarrett was the only child among six hundred adults. The many people who came over to his table to congratulate him made him feel good, but he had his eye on Father Nguyen, who was working the room like a used car salesman, stopping at every table. Jarrett made a mental note to add a couple of lines to his acceptance speech.

When the program began, the lights dimmed and everyone turned their attention to Bishop Kendrick Williams. One by one, he called the winners to the podium, telling how their good works exemplified the love of God. The honorees included a medical missionary to Guatemala and a couple who had opened their home to more than twenty foster children.

"They were truly holy people who lived by the Bible every day," Jennifer said.

After a couple of hours, it finally came time to present Jarrett his award. A slide presentation played out, showing Jarrett at home with his family and at the children's hospital pushing The Joy Cart.

When the lights came back up, Jarrett stepped up to the microphone to the thunderous applause he had become accustomed to. He accepted the award, shook the Bishop's hand, and posed for a photograph.

And then, his mother said, he decided to do a standup routine.

"As long as I'm up here, I have a few things I want to take care of," Jarrett said.

Oh no, thought Jennifer. She wondered where her son's speech was headed.

"Please, Jarrett," she said to herself. "These are church people. This is a pious occasion. Don't get silly."

But Jarrett wanted to roast his friend in the priesthood.

"Do you know what it's like trying to serve mass with Father Linh?" Jarrett asked the crowd. "He makes these little twitches with his head, left and right, and I can never figure out what he wants me to do."

Those in the crowd from Jarrett's parish laughed. They were familiar with Nguyen's mannerisms.

"And people worry about my health, but they should worry about Father Linh. Did you see how he was going from table to table tonight, toasting everybody with wine? He must've put away quite a few bottles. I'm worried about *his* health."

The Father shook his finger at Jarrett and smiled. The crowd roared.

Then Jarrett thanked his parents and other family members for all they had done to support his project. He asked them to stand from their table in the right corner of the room.

"If you get a blinding glare from over there, that's my Granny Jeanne. She always has sequins on."

Again, the crowd laughed. Jarrett's grandmother was mortified. She didn't think he was giving the proper acceptance speech for such a highly religious ceremony.

Jennifer worried about that, too, until the benediction was delivered and people started to move toward the door.

"Many people came over and thanked Jarrett for lightening the mood," she said. "And the Bishop had laughed as loudly as anyone in the room had. So I guess it was O.K. Maybe Jarrett had sat through too many solemn speeches that night and just had to burn up some energy."

No matter what the occasion, Jarrett always seemed to steal the show. And his family believed the axiom that laughter is good medicine. Plus, he couldn't wait to go to church again. Maybe he just wanted to get more material to use against Father Linh. But, whatever his motivation, his mother knew that church was good for him.

35

Oprah

Over the years, Jarrett had impressed more and more journalists with his gentle spirit, his speaking abilities, and his quotable quotes. He was a good story, there was no doubt about it.

One reporter who never forgot the young man was Melinda Morrison, who had interviewed him while working at WHAS-TV in Louisville.

"Melinda kept up with us through e-mail," Jennifer said. "She wasn't like so many reporters who pass through your life once and you never see them again. She checked in often to get an update on Jarrett's condition."

My co-anchor at WDKY developed the same kind of relationship. Jennifer Nime understood Melinda's affection. "Jarrett was just one of those people you couldn't get out of your mind once you met him," she said.

My on-air partner, who was single then, often found that Jarrett was a good Saturday night date. She took him to movies and to dinner many times. I teased her about "liking them young."

No doubt, Melinda would have done the same thing had she lived closer. By the beginning of 2000, she had moved back to her native Seattle to do freelance work. Part of her work included producing segments for talk show queen Oprah Winfrey.

Melinda worked for months to try to convince the Oprah producers to do a segment about Jarrett.

"I fell in love with the kid the first time I met him," Melinda said. "He was magic. I saw him healing kids as he went room to room with his Joy Cart—not curing them, but healing their broken spirits."

In November, the time was right. The show was a few months into a project called "Remembering Your Spirit," which was a series of videotaped reports about people who were making a difference in the world. It included stories about people who overcame all sorts of obstacles from discrimination to medical hardships and incredible financial burdens.

Melinda pitched the story to producers in Chicago when they called her looking for ideas for a segment on medical miracles.

"I had one day to get on a plane and get to Kentucky," she said. "I called Jarrett's mother and apologized for the short notice. But I was determined to get there and get it done."

She contracted with a production crew from Cincinnati and showed up at UK Children's Hospital November 3, 2000.

Melinda scoped out the hospital and made small talk with the Mynears and hospital public relations staff as she waited for the crew to arrive. More than an hour passed, and she began to stress out. It was a Friday afternoon. Many of the children were about to be released for the weekend. She wanted to get a lot of video of Jarrett passing out toys, but if the crew didn't hurry up, there wouldn't be many kids to put on camera. Melinda wanted this story to be just right, and it was off to a bad start.

At last, the crew pulled into the hospital's loading zone. The driver apologized, telling Melinda how he had gotten lost.

But she barely heard the words. She quickly rushed the crew to the hospital's playroom and supervised while it set up lights, tested camera angles, and did microphone checks.

At last, when it seemed everything was working, Melinda called Jennifer and Jarrett in to do an interview.

Just as she began to ask a question, the sound of jackhammers pierced the air. The hospital was in the middle of a major renovation.

"Stop!" Melinda shouted frantically. "We can't do the interview with all that noise in the background."

When the racket died down, Melinda resumed the interview and, as she put it, Jarrett gave phenomenal answers. But before he could complete his thoughts, the hammering began again.

"Jarrett would give me a perfect sound bite, and I would have to do it over and over," she said. Frustration got the best of her.

She excused herself and went to find the hospital's public relations person. That set off a chain of events that took another hour to resolve. The university had to make a series of calls to get the construction crews to stop for a few minutes. Time is money, and it is no easy task to inject a manmade (or in this case, womanmade) delay into the work schedule of state-paid contractors.

"By that time, I was begging parents to hold their kids there for a little while longer," she said. "Most of them understood it was a big deal to be on *The Oprah Winfrey Show*, so they were quite nice about it."

As she was about to wave the white flag of surrender, the jackhammers fell silent.

Later, everyone at the hospital would joke about how only Jarrett could bring construction to a halt. Sick people had to listen to the noise every day and would have no doubt loved to have pulled the plug on the ruckus many times, but only this eleven-year-old boy had actually been able to do it.

Melinda conducted a poignant interview. She still remembers the last thing Jarrett said while the cameras were rolling.

"I don't know how much longer I'll be here," he said, without a hint of drama. "But I hope the kids will remember that I did something nice for them and they'll do something kind for someone in their life."

Tears welled up in Melinda's eyes. It was like she had been hit by one of those jackhammers on the other side of the wall. She turned and looked at the camera operator, who was also wiping the corner of his eyes.

When the story aired exactly a week later, no one could have known it was a rush job. It was beautifully done and, despite all the chaos, Jarrett's personality shone through. Melinda didn't see the show, and she knew Oprah wouldn't see the segment until it played in front of her on live TV. She was in an airport as the show ended. Her cell phone rang and a producer in Chicago said simply, "You made the boss cry."

As the show went off the air, the last thing viewers saw was Jarrett's smiling face. The closing credits included his e-mail address.

Melinda decided after the show that she wanted to help Jarrett's dream of expansion come true. Many people had talked about forming their own Joy

Carts, but none had gotten off the ground on a regular schedule.

"I just couldn't get it out of my mind," she said. "I thought, 'This is something I can do. I have the complete power to do what Jarrett is asking.'"

Within days, she had presented a business proposal to the Seattle Children's Hospital—an idea it accepted immediately.

"Melinda called us now and again and said, 'I'm serious about this. I want to do it here in Seattle,'" Jennifer said. "We thought that was a nice idea, but we really didn't put much stock in it."

They soon learned they had underestimated the wrong person.

36

"You've Got Mail"

The phone rang at the Mynear household all evening after the taped piece ran on Oprah. Just as with the Rosie O'Donnell appearances, friends and relatives wanted to call to congratulate Jarrett on his performance. No one in the family got around to checking their e-mail that night.

But the next day, when Jennifer logged on to her AOL account, the familiar digitized voice informed her: "You've Got Mail."

Boy, did she ever. The page was full, and as she scrolled down, it just seemed to go on and on. Hundreds of messages filled the in-box. She didn't recognize the account names of the senders. They were all Oprah viewers who had jotted down the address as the show went off the air.

She called Jarrett into the room so he could see the instantaneous response.

"Oh my gosh, Mom," Jarrett said. "How are we going to read all that?"

After they looked at the first five or six messages, they made a decision.

"We have to respond to these," Jennifer said. "All of them. These people were nice enough to say these things; we can't ignore them."

She thought they would just take a few at a time. They crafted a form letter of sorts to send en masse, but it became apparent that wasn't always the appropriate response.

"Many of the writers had specific questions, and quite a few of them wanted to know how they could start their own toy carts," Jennifer said. "And many of them wanted to know more about Jarrett's cancer, saying they had a child or a relative who had just been diagnosed with Ewing's and were at a loss for information."

For the rest of the week, Doug and Jennifer and Jarrett all spent time answering the e-mail. But the new messages were coming in faster than they could clear the old ones. When the count reached 1,500, the family decided it needed help.

Jennifer mentioned the volume of response to Jarrett's computer lab instructor. Jarrett was one of the star pupils in STLP, the Student Technology Leadership Program. The group was made up of several students who were junior computer wizards. These kids set up networks within the school and taught other students how to use the advanced functions on the computers. The sixth-, seventh- and eighth-graders were often called to troubleshoot problems for teachers in the classroom.

Jarrett had been interested in computers since he was eighteen months old. Long before he reached school age, he would sit in Doug's lap and they would play games, write programs, and surf the web together.

"Jarrett definitely got that from his dad," Jennifer said. "I can't do much beyond the basics."

Jarrett's lab instructor suggested working the Oprah responses into the curriculum for the STLP students. The Mynears were glad to take her up on the offer.

The Mynears forwarded the e-mail to the school's computer lab, and the students took the challenge to respond to the letters and ran with it. They set up address books, wrote several reply letters to fit different situations, and even cross-referenced responses. For example, if three people in central Ohio expressed an interest in starting a toy cart, the students got them in contact with each other.

"It was a tremendous help to us," Jennifer said. "Of course, when they agreed to do it, I'm not sure they realized the letters would keep coming."

Hundreds more letters were forwarded from the Oprah staff—letters that had gone to them instead of directly to the Mynears.

"I want to emphasize that we read every letter and every message," Jennifer said. "We just let the students help respond. People have a right to know their message got to us. When they were of a more personal nature, I responded personally."

Jarrett had hundreds of the messages printed out and he kept them in binders. If he ever had doubts about the impact of his project, they vanished when he read the e-mail:

What an awesome young man you are! I am a mother of three. I live in a small town in Texas. I feel pretty confident we could get the donations for this but my question to you is this: Could we name our cart after you?

****

I am a 34 yr. old wife and mother and just want to tell you that God is so very proud of you. Your life is a wonderful example of how we all should live.

****

Hey there, we think you are the best. Because of you we are looking into starting a joy cart ourselves here in Florida. We honor your spirit!!

****

I am 24 years old and I live alone in a single bedroom apartment in Edmonton, Alberta, Canada. I don't have very much but I have decided to help you. I thought at first I would send money, but I don't think that would be enough. Instead, I will help the kids that are here. Maybe a teddy bear given to a child will help them fight.

****

I have been feeling sorry for myself because I have been laid off for over 2.5 months. When I saw your story today, I was just lying in bed. When I listened to you speak, hearing your sensitivity and wisdom brought me to tears.

On Monday when the various business offices open, I am going to check into starting a toy cart or at least volunteering my time at the local children's hospital. I feel like you have given this 38-year-old person a new lease on life.

****

My heart swelled to see today's Oprah show. I am sending $100 and hope that you can make a few children smile. I also intend to inquire as to whether there is an opportunity to have a Jarrett's cart in our local hospital here in New Jersey.

****

Have you ever considered that you are a role model for several adults? Well, it's true. Thanks for warming my heart.

****

Hi there Jarrett—

Today I saw you on Oprah. Your outlook and kindness made me cry. Even my 6-year-old little boy said "Wow, what a nice kid." Keep up the great work!

****

I consider myself your #1 fan, and even though I only saw you on TV a few minutes ago, you are my favorite person in the world besides my family, of course.

****

Hey Jarrett: Don't know if you remember me, but I was with you the day we all visited the White House, met Buddy, and got pushed aside as President Clinton strolled by. My whole company decided to dedicate this day to you and together focus our energies on your speedy recovery. One of the guys even asked (after I told him how cool you were) if we could put you in one of our movies. Let's just say the vote was a big unanimous YES!

So get better soon. We'll get you out here and put that smile of yours in front of the camera!

Your buddy (not the dog),

Corbin Bernsen

The ways people thought of to help astounded the Mynears. Several families made it their Christmas project to put extra gifts around the tree marked for "Jarrett's Joy Cart."

ACE Insurance Company in their town of Nicholasville organized a "poker run," in which nearly a hundred motorcyclists traveled to several checkpoints, picking up a different playing card at each stop. At the end of the ride, the best hand won a prize. Jarrett strapped on a helmet and rode on the back of a Harley Davidson with one of the organizers. All of the proceeds went to The Joy Cart.

The local Goody's department store sponsored a car show in its parking lot. Entry fees went to the hospital.

Insight Communications, the Lexington cable company, offered free installation for a month to any customer who would donate a new toy or $10 to The Joy Cart. It took in $8,000 and four hundred toys.

And the Lexington Rotary Club invited the Mynears to a meeting, saying the endowment committee wanted to make a donation. The family expected maybe a few hundred dollars. Jarrett almost fell over when the committee president handed him an oversized check for $20,000. The symbolic check represented the club's pledge to allocate money for years to come.

One Nicholasville man donated more than six hundred Beanie Babies. Clarence Rogers had bought, sold, and collected the squeezable stuffed animals for years.

"The hobby had gotten out of hand," Rogers told a local newspaper reporter. Hundreds of the toys were left over from McDonald's Happy Meal boxes. Rogers said the family's two German shepherds helped eat a lot of hamburgers when the collection was being built up. "When we heard about The Joy Cart, we knew exactly what to do with the toys. Children at the hospital will enjoy them more than we do."

That was the first time Jarrett could count dogs among his growing list of donors.

37

A Ton of Bricks

During the fall of 2000, Jarrett was fitted with a new prosthesis—his fourth. It took him a month or so to feel comfortable with it as he adjusted to the new length and the minor differences in the tension and flexibility in the knee joint.

He began to complain off and on that October about back pain and soreness in his hip, but his parents believed that was still just part of getting used to the new leg. They had been told to expect some soreness for quite a while as Jarrett's spine adjusted to his new stance.

"I also noticed he was beginning to lose weight again," Jennifer said. "But appetite had always been as issue with Jarrett. It was something that came and went."

Still, as they went to the hospital in November for Jarrett's next scheduled round of bone scans, Jennifer had a bad feeling. Things had been going better than they probably had a right to expect them to for a long time. It had been more than two years since his bone marrow transplant. His spirit had been buoyed by the Oprah exposure just a few days before.

"There were no glaring red flags as we went to the hospital that day," she said. "Again, it was just part of the routine."

Her good friend Kathy Tabb went too, planning to join them for a nice lunch once the tests were completed.

Jarrett went in for a CAT scan first.

"The technicians had always been wonderful," Jennifer said. "They would chitchat and joke around and make us feel at ease."

But this day was different. The technicians seemed especially quiet when they did the scans, and from time to time they would whisper something, obviously trying to keep their voices low enough so Jennifer could not hear them.

"They had never avoided me before, but I could tell they knew something was wrong."

She didn't confront them then, but she began to feel sick to her stomach. Her strong intuition told her she had better brace herself for bad news. Other mothers may have demanded that the technicians stop whispering and tell them what they were seeing on their monitors, but Jennifer was not in any hurry to hear what had them concerned. She kept watching for some sign of hope—a smile, relaxed facial muscles, a freeing sigh—anything that could indicate her fears were unfounded.

The scans were taken away for Dr. Martha Greenwood to read.

"She always made it a point to talk to Jarrett when we went in for tests," Jennifer said. "But that day, she made herself scarce. I asked when she would come in to see us, and they kept telling me she was too busy; she had no time to talk."

Jennifer looked at Kathy and told her she was getting bad vibes. Kathy tried to reassure Jennifer that it was too early to be worried. She fibbed when she said she didn't get the impression the technicians were avoiding them.

"They're just busier than usual today," Kathy said. But deep down, Kathy had the same gut feeling that bad news was brewing.

Then, the staffers took Jarrett to a different table for a bone scan.

"I got the same evasive looks and when I asked how it was going, I got vague answers," Jennifer said.

Time crept, but eventually a nurse called Jennifer into the hall and told her Dr. Greenwood wanted to talk to her. The walk to the doctor's station seemed like a trip to the gallows.

Dr. Greenwood had a grim look on her face as she got straight to the point. She told Jennifer cancer had invaded Jarrett's skeleton in the spine.

"I won't lie to you," the doctor said. "It's bad. You may want to get Doug here while we study the scans."

Once again, Jennifer felt as though she had been hit by the proverbial ton of bricks, with a force as strong as the one she absorbed the first time she was told her toddler had cancer at age two-and-a-half.

"It was probably even worse this time," Jennifer said. "The first time, there was naiveté on our part. Now, I really knew what he could be facing."

A technician took her into a private office so she could call her husband. She broke down in tears and had trouble composing her thoughts as she punched in Doug's phone number.

Outside the office, Kathy cried and several of the nurses mopped their own tears. It seemed that entire wing of the hospital was cloaked in sadness as the word spread. None of the nurses knew what to do to make it better. If it would have helped to throw a chair or let out a chorus of primal screams, they would have done it. Jarrett was everybody's little buddy, and now it appeared their favorite patient was "too far gone." Maybe they were feeling as sorry for themselves as they were for him. They could not imagine not having Jarrett around anymore.

When Doug arrived, Chief Pediatric Oncologist Dr. Jeffrey Moscow joined them to discuss the CAT scan. It showed at least twelve small tumors on Jarrett's liver and a softball-sized tumor clinging to the right side of his abdomen. They could see how the largest tumor was squeezing Jarrett's stomach outward.

Jarrett had lost more weight than his parents realized. The swollen stomach had fooled them.

"Basically, he had no stomach left," Jennifer said. "It was almost all tumor. The doctors couldn't understand how he had been eating at all."

The tumors had seemed to come so suddenly. A check back at a bone scan three months earlier did show some dark marks on the spine. That had been attributed to the "wear and tear" of Jarrett's shifting posture as he adjusted to his new leg.

The doctors did a biopsy to confirm whether this was another case of Ewing's sarcoma. It was. The disease proved once again how malicious it could be. It had stayed dormant and hidden for four years, but it refused to go away for good.

38
Something to Say

The bad news could not keep Jarrett from his next public appearance. If anything, it made him more determined to find an audience.

He had been asked to join the Kentucky delegation on the President's Cancer Panel, a conference organized by the National Cancer Institute. The institute set up a series of meetings around the country to gather information to be presented to President George W. Bush and members of Congress.

Jarrett was the only child asked to participate. The meeting in Nashville would include presentations by health care professionals from eight southern states, Puerto Rico, and the U.S. Virgin Islands.

It was scheduled for November 16th and 17th, just a week after the devastating diagnosis.

"I thought about calling the Kentucky leaders and telling them to get another representative," Jennifer said. "But Jarrett insisted on going. He had done his homework. He had interviewed Dr. Moscow. He felt he had something to say that the President needed to hear."

Jarrett was concerned that if he didn't go, there would be no children on the panel. And he truly believed children should have a voice.

The topic was equity in insurance coverage. Jarrett found out from Dr. Moscow that a lot of the children at the UK Hospital were on Medicaid. Many of them received more than one type of chemotherapy per day, but Medicaid would only pay for one daily treatment.

Jennifer helped Jarrett write his speech, using her son's notes.

The second day of the conference at Vanderbilt University was Kentucky's day to make a presentation. The delegation would get one hour to speak that morning. Jarrett sat on the dais with four other guests, including the director of the Markey Cancer Center and a colorectal surgeon from Louisville.

Each of the four spoke ahead of Jarrett. The woman who addressed the panel just before Jarrett's turn talked about getting malignant melanoma in October 1986, breast cancer in her left side in October 1994, and breast cancer on the right in October 1996.

"So, you see, I don't like the month of October at all," she said.

When Jarrett was introduced, the panel's chairman set a microphone at the table for him. He was too small to go to the podium.

He began, as usual, looking totally relaxed.

"Like Ms. Farris was saying, her bad month is October. Mine is September," he began. "Three of my diagnoses have been in September, all around the same date."

That wasn't in the script.

Jennifer became nervous. She didn't want him to ad-lib. From her seat in the audience, she began waving a copy of his speech, pointing at it frantically.

Jarrett nodded his acknowledgement and began to read his prepared remarks.

Jennifer sat back, breathing easier. Doug patted her hand, indicating things would be O.K.

Jarrett told the audience how he had just been re-diagnosed a week before and how he was prepared to go another round with cancer.

"Even though I'm not feeling well, it's important for me that you hear about my concern for the cancer patients of Kentucky, especially the children.

"As you can imagine, my family and I have met hundreds of pediatric patients over the years. And one of the most important things we've learned is that to get through this, you have to have a good system to meet *all* the needs of the patients and their families, not just the medical ones.

"Many of the families would be better able to cope with the diagnoses, treatments, and all the other things that follow if they had a good psychological support system. We have seen families break apart because of the stress of long hospitalizations and the uncertainty of their children's illnesses.

"Families with private insurance rarely find that coverage is offered for services to help them learn to cope with the stresses cancer brings into a family, especially one where there are siblings. For those in Kentucky with public insurance, these services are typically not available either.

"Cancer not only brings health worries, but it brings financial pressures and emotional stresses as well. I know, firsthand, the importance of having a positive, healthy attitude and knowing that my family is beside me all the way."

Jarrett went on to address the Medicaid issue and the fact that multiple daily chemo treatments were not covered.

"Medicaid only pays for one of those treatments. The rest are given, as they should be, but payment comes from the pool of money used to run and staff the pediatric oncology department.

"Our hospital doesn't have enough nurses or doctors because the money is being used to cover chemotherapy and its administration, as well as other procedures, since Kentucky's Medicaid doesn't. This means the pediatric patients suffer because of low staffing."

Then Jarrett eloquently told the panel about his late friend C. B. Wolford. Jarrett said there was a real problem with a delay of diagnoses for children who lived in rural areas.

"C. B. didn't even have a fighting chance to battle his cancer because doctors at home kept telling his parents that he was having growing pains and was just getting lazy when he complained of being very sore and very tired. A CAT scan clearly showed a large tumor in his lung, but it was not identified at that time. The doctor who dealt with C. B. told his mother that he was probably developing breast tissue due to puberty. He said that he had a little more than most boys, but he would be fine.

"*Where* you live in a state shouldn't be a factor in how quickly you are diagnosed and provided with cutting-edge treatment and choices."

As he was about to close, Jarrett looked up from his script.

"Mom, if you're taking a picture, the shutter is closed."

Jennifer just shook her head. But she looked at her camera and he was right. The audience laughed. Jennifer's face turned red.

Then he wrapped things up, not immodestly, by saying, "I'm a hard act to follow. I guess that's why they put me at the end of the line."

There wasn't a speaker on the program who would deny it, as the audience responded with a standing ovation.

39

Downhill

In the days that followed, Dr. Moscow talked to the Mynears about a clinical trial for immuno-therapy that was starting at the National Institutes for Health (NIH). That would mean a series of vaccines. He told them it might be too late for conventional treatment. This could possibly be Jarrett's only glimmer of hope.

So, in mid-December the family went once again to yet another unfamiliar hospital, the research center in Bethesda, Maryland. If it was grasping at straws, so be it. Give them a handful. Because of Jarrett's determination, "giving up" was a phrase that had long ago been wiped out of their vocabulary.

In the week before they made the trip, Jarrett's condition deteriorated rapidly. The pain in his spine and abdomen grew much worse, and he took large amounts of pain medication. He stopped wearing his artificial leg and stayed in a wheelchair most of his waking hours.

"The Ewing's came in bursts," his mother said. "It broke through two vertebrae in his neck. He couldn't hold his head up as we went into a meeting with the protocol chairman at the hospital in Maryland."

The doctors there had Jarrett admitted immediately. They placed him under an around-the-clock neurological watch, concerned he could be paralyzed if there were any more strain on his neck.

The next day, the doctors stood over Jarrett's bed and told his family he needed twenty more days of radiation on the two main tumor sites on his spine.

"At that point, Jarrett rolled over, curled up into a ball, and tuned everybody out," his mother said. "He didn't want to hear that he wasn't going anywhere."

Again, Christmas was just around the corner, and the boy could not stand the thought of not being home for the holiday.

Another day passed, and the radiologists were in disagreement about the safety of moving Jarrett. Some believed they could get him stabilized in a couple of days and allow him to return to Kentucky for the radiation. Others thought he should stay put.

Dr. Moscow consulted with the NIH doctors over the telephone and assured them they could take care of Jarrett at UK. They agreed on three days of radiation in Maryland, coupled with a dose of steroids to reduce the swelling in the spinal column.

"The doctors at NIH were very methodical," Jennifer said. "They took great care to make sure he could travel. They checked his response to the radiation every day and decided he was O.K. to fly."

So on the evening of the third treatment, Doug and Jennifer bundled their children in warm jackets and got on a plane home. Jarrett was extremely weak. His family had seen him go downhill rapidly that week.

"We weren't sure if it was stress, fatigue, or anxiety," his mother said. "But we knew we had to get his spirits up. Getting home for Christmas was part of that strategy."

Their plane touched down in Louisville late that night, and they made the ninety-minute drive home. They were due at the UK Children's Hospital at 7:30 A.M. for a radiation treatment.

"We were exhausted," Jennifer said. "But it was worth it to be back home."

The radiation continued for the next three weeks, five days a week, attacking those two tumor sites on the spine. The tumor on the abdomen was much too large to irradiate. The doctors were still wondering what to do about it. They couldn't just cut it out. They didn't know exactly how it was connected to other organs, and an operation could have caused severe bleeding.

They spent Christmas Eve at their home with Doug's family and made the traditional visit to Granny Jeanne's house on Christmas Day. All of the relatives who came to either house tried to act as if nothing had changed.

"But it was very melancholy," Jennifer said. "We had trouble putting on a happy face. We all knew things had never been this bad with Jarrett. He was on so much pain medication he could barely stay awake at times."

The steroids had changed his mood. The young boy who never seemed to get down about his condition now had times when he was short-tempered and withdrawn.

He sat at the holiday dinner table that was covered with casseroles, vegetables, and sweets and tried to take a bite of his favorite dishes.

"He wanted to eat so badly," Jennifer said. "But he'd take one bite and sit there with tears in his eyes. It made him feel full and bloated."

His circumstances were taking a physiological toll on Jarrett.

In the week that followed, Jennifer suspended all efforts to keep Jarrett current with his schoolwork. He couldn't go to school, and she didn't even try to put textbooks or homework in front of him. That was something she had never ignored before.

"He was just too sick to keep his mind on anything," she said. "Some days he would be overdosed and in a stupor."

It upset Jarrett to have those feelings of disorientation. He tried not to take the pain medications because he didn't like the way they made him feel. But pain almost always won out.

Jarrett's liver was not clearing out the way it should. One tumor blocked his bile duct, causing toxins to back up into his body. At times he could not go to the bathroom at all. His throat became constricted, making it almost impossible to swallow. Sometimes he spit up blood or it showed up in his urine. Even though two inches of snow covered the ground outside Jarrett's window, everything seemed dark to the Mynears.

Jarrett now looked jaundiced and bloated. He felt horrible, and the doctors wanted desperately to ease the pain. Dr. Moscow talked with a cardiologist about using a stent to open Jarrett's bile duct to give him some relief, and they both agreed it was worth a try. When Jarrett showed up at the hospital for the procedure, a doctor his family hadn't seen before came into the room, took Jarrett's hand and said, "I know who you are, and I want you to know what an honor it is for me to try to help you."

Once Jarrett was unconscious, the doctor put a wire down his throat all the way to the spot on his bile duct. The idea was to then slide the stent down that wire into the position where the tumor was pressing on the bile duct. The family waited just outside the procedure room for well over an hour, wondering why it was taking so long.

Finally, a nurse came out. There was strain on her face and in her voice as she told the family the doctor was having trouble getting the stent in place because of the size of the tumor. He wanted their permission to try again while Jarrett was still under anesthesia. So they waited for what seemed like another hour.

"At last, the doctor came out," Jennifer recalled. "His face was as white as his coat, and he had tears in his eyes. We all thought Jarrett had died."

But instead, the doctor had good news—the kind that sends shivers down your spine.

He said, "I just witnessed a miracle. I had been trying and trying to work that stent into place, and it just wouldn't cooperate. I put my head down and said, 'God, you've got to help me.'"

He told the Mynears he had the end of the wire and the stent in his hand as he said that little prayer, and when he let go of it, the stent slid right into the duct as if guided by an invisible hand and the bile started flowing immediately.

"We all started crying," Jennifer said. "When Jarrett came into the room, he was a different child. He was talkative, and you could tell he felt so much better. It had been instant relief. By the next day, his eyes and complexion no longer looked yellow. He had his energy back."

When the radiation regimen ended, Dr. Moscow decided to attack the abdominal tumor with a combination of two types of chemotherapy that had worked for Jarrett at separate times. It was a shot in the dark whether the two would enhance each other's effectiveness.

As Dr. Moscow discussed his plan with Jennifer during an office visit, Jarrett began to ask questions. It was clear he needed things laid out in black and white.

"I nodded to Dr. Moscow, indicating it was O.K. to be straight with Jarrett," his mother said. "We had always been honest with him, and he knew things were getting worse every day. There was no need to sugarcoat it for him."

But there is no easy way to tell a child he is probably going to die. Dr. Moscow looked Jarrett straight in the eyes and told him the severity of the situation and how the cancer had invaded his liver, pancreas and skeleton.

"The choices are limited, Jarrett," the doctor said. "As you know, Ewing's is a smart cancer, and it may have developed immunity to the chemo we want to use. We just don't know if it will work."

Jarrett dropped his head, and tears flowed as if a spigot had been opened. Jennifer lost her composure, and Dr. Moscow excused himself.

The boy climbed onto his mother's lap, and they held each other in silence for several minutes.

Then Jarrett raised his head, wiped his tears with the back of his hand, and looked at his mother.

"It's going to be all right," he said. "I've done this before, and I can do it again. It's going to be all right."

"It's going to be all right." He repeated it again, and he patted his mother on the back.

"I reminded him that parents are the ones who are supposed to keep it together in these situations," Jennifer said, amazed that her son was the one who was doing the consoling.

"I know, Mom, but I'm better at it than you," Jarrett said, forcing a smile.

A couple of the nurses stood at their work station just around the corner, including Anne Hoskins, who had worked at the clinic twenty-five years and had tended to Jarrett since his first day there. The nurses huddled together and shared the sorrow, as they tried to muffle their crying.

Later, Nurse Anne told Jarrett she felt like kicking the wall when she heard he had been diagnosed with cancer again.

"Anne," Jarrett replied, "That would just be wasting energy that could be used for something positive."

Anne tried to fill her head with positive thoughts. It wasn't difficult to think of things about Jarrett that made her laugh. She remembered the time he came out of the chemo room with blood all over his face.

"We were all about to faint," Anne said. "It looked like something had gone terribly wrong. Then he started laughing. It was all fake. He had painted himself with something he had gotten out of a Halloween makeup kit."

And she recalled how Jarrett had learned to mimic the noises the IV machines made.

"He could imitate the beeping sounds perfectly," she said. "As soon as a nurse would leave the room, he'd start in—'beep . . . beep'—and we'd come running, thinking it was time to change the fluids. Everyone else in the room would break out laughing. It would drive us crazy, running back and forth."

It was that spirit that kept her upbeat about a potentially-depressing job.

Jarrett asked his mother to bring Dr. Moscow back into the room.

"Tell me again what the options are," he asked the doctor.

"We can either take the aggressive route and try to slow the cancer down, or we can give you medications to make sure you're comfortable," Moscow said.

"The chemo would be harsh and could make you really sick. To be honest, Jarrett, it could affect your quality of life."

Jarrett looked at Dr. Moscow, squarely and firmly. He made sure there was eye contact.

"You give me the chemo, and I'll be fine," he said.

"I'm not going to lie to you," Moscow said. "This is hard-core chemo."

"It's not my time to go," Jarrett replied. "You give me the chemo, and I'll take care of the rest of it."

And that was that.

Jarrett went home that day, with skin and eyes yellowed with jaundice once again, skinny arms and a distended stomach that made him look like one of the starving children you see in drought-ravaged Third World countries. But, even in that state, he showed strength.

"After he made his choices, he moved on," Dr. Moscow said. "I had many tough conversations with him. But the next thing you'd know, he'd be playing video games. We all wish we could dispatch the great issues in our life with such ease."

When Jarrett showed up to begin the round of chemotherapy, the doctors ordered yet another CAT scan. His mother described the image of his stomach as "a squashed file folder." The tumor took up all the space.

For the first few days, the doctors had Jarrett on low doses. He handled it well so they gradually pushed the treatments to full strength. But Jarrett was a long way from the vibrant child he was known to be.

Many of the regular patients at the pediatric clinic refused to go into the treatment room when Jarrett was there.

"It hurt them too badly to see Jarrett in that shape," Jennifer said. "One boy stayed in the waiting room and got his chemo treatments there."

Each day when Jennifer wheeled Jarrett into the clinic, she made sure not to make eye contact with Anne and some of the other nurses. Just a glance could make them all fall apart, and Jarrett did not need to see any more tears.

One day in early February, Kathy Tabb sat with Jarrett as he got his treatment. Jennifer was away on an errand.

He told Kathy he wanted to do something special for his mother for Valentine's Day. Kathy thought about it for a moment and then asked Jarrett if he would like to paint ceramics.

He thought that was a good idea, so Kathy arranged to take him to The Mad Potter—a shop that lets customers put their own designs on mugs, plates and bowls before they are glazed and fired.

"He was really sick when I took him there. He had been spitting up blood and felt miserable, but he insisted on going ahead with it," Kathy said.

As they scanned the shelves at the store, Jarrett seemed to take forever to pick out something to paint. He was slower than some of the kids who became overwhelmed when they were invited to get something off The Joy Cart.

Finally, he chose a coffee mug.

Kathy and Jarrett sat at the wooden table, with more than a dozen colors of paint opened in front of them. Jarrett moved slowly and carefully, painting hearts and flowers around the sides of the mug.

Then he took a brush and covered the entire palm of his hand with blue paint.

"Jarrett, you're making a mess!" Kathy said. "You're going to get paint all over your mug."

"I know," he said softly.

Then he wrapped his entire hand around the mug and grasped it firmly.

When he pulled his hand away, there was a perfect imprint of his hand.

"I want Mom to always be able to hold my hand," he said. "All she'll have to do is pick up this mug and I'll be with her."

Tears welled up in Kathy's eyes. It was heart-wrenching. She couldn't believe he had come up with such a profound idea.

Jennifer had the same reaction when Jarrett presented the gift to her a week later. That multi-colored mug instantly became the most precious piece in the china cabinet.

By the end of February, Jarrett started to eat more solid foods, and he began to get out of the wheelchair more. He didn't use the prosthesis much. He accepted being carried.

In mid-March, the doctors did another CAT scan and an MRI, and both showed some shrinkage of the tumor.

"Not anything tremendous, mind you," said Jennifer. "It was just a matter of millimeters. But it was in the right direction."

Two more weeks passed, and the family could tell Jarrett was feeling better. The jaundice went away, as did the swelling in his stomach.

As always, his parents were concerned about his emotional well-being. "We had learned that had a lot to do with how he did physically," Jennifer said.

So, again they allowed him to accept invitations and to be reintroduced to the active social life to which he had been accustomed.

Terry Hagan often showed up with his pickup to take Jarrett to a movie. He would throw the wheelchair in the back, hoist Jarrett in the cab, and off they would go. Sometimes they would just go to Terry's house to watch a rented movie on his VCR. Once they took a trip to Fort Knox. As a retired Army reservist, Terry had connections. Jarrett had a grand time climbing over the tanks and sitting in an Apache helicopter.

Three other kids went on the trip, too, which turned into a twelve-hour day.

"There wasn't a minute when one of them wasn't talking," Terry remembered. "When we went into the military museum, Jarrett started teaching class—telling the others all about the helmets, the survival kits, and the firepower of the weapons. You would have never known he was sick."

Jennifer's brother Christopher organized similar outings, hauling his nephew off to go fishing, watch hockey games, or eat at ice cream parlors.

And several Lexington police officers took Jarrett under their wings as a little brother, often taking him on field trips so he could see their vehicles and crime-fighting tools up close.

"I'd hold my breath every time," Jennifer admitted. She knew Jarrett did not feel well, but he refused to be homebound.

The police department printed thousands of collectible cards that pictured officers kids may see in the community—those who worked with dogs or rode bicycles, motorcycles, and horses. The idea was to pass them out in schools and on playgrounds to make children feel comfortable around police. An additional trading card showed up in the deck in the spring of 2001. The police made Jarrett an honorary member of the force and featured him on a card.

"It was good for him to have all these distractions," Jennifer said.

The chemo was adding quantity to his life. His parents wanted to be sure there was quality, too.

40

Faith

Robin Silverman says she has spent more than thirty years looking for the good in people. The inspirational author from Grand Forks, North Dakota, collects stories of ordinary people who do extraordinary things. It was just a matter of time before she discovered Jarrett.

After a speech for a rotary club in Texas, a man in the audience told Robin about Taryn Pream, a teenager from Thief River Falls, Minnesota. In 1998, Taryn became the victim of Internet harassment. She received disturbing e-mail messages that said things such as "I am your worst nightmare" and "Your troubles are just beginning." Fear overtook her, and her grades slipped dramatically over several weeks as the e-mail kept coming. But the local sheriff's department tracked down the culprit, one of Taryn's classmates, and sentenced him to one hundred hours of community service. Had he been an adult, he would have faced jail time.

Taryn turned the negative into a positive, developing brochures and an educational program for other teens to tell them how to use the Internet safely—warning them about stalkers in the chat rooms and the consequences of sending threats through cyberspace.

Robin contacted Taryn, hoping to tell her story in an upcoming book entitled *Something Wonderful is About to Happen*. Taryn was glad to tell her story; she also told Silverman she had a friend the author should know about. That friend was Jarrett Mynear, whom Taryn had met as a fellow winner of the Prudential Spirit of Community Awards.

"All I knew about when I picked up the phone was The Joy Cart," Robin said. "But as I talked to Jarrett's mother on the phone, I quickly learned about his latest diagnosis, and I felt a sense of urgency and helplessness."

Robin asked Jennifer if she believed in the power of prayer.

"That's always been an important thing to us," Jennifer said. "It gets us through a lot of dark days."

Robin, who had really just begun to know about this family and its complicated journey, felt compelled to write a prayer for Jarrett.

She told Jennifer how her mother-in-law had been given six hours to live, as she lay in a bed comatose and on life-support.

"We were told to gather the family," Robin said. "She wasn't expected to make it through the night."

But as she stood over the bed, the family's rabbi came in and told her how the congregation was praying for her mother-in-law. A few minutes later, a Catholic priest stopped by and said he would be praying. And within the hour, the hospital's Protestant chaplain popped his head into the room to say the same thing.

Robin's mother-in-law made a full recovery, and Robin became convinced it was because of the prayers.

"The doctors were baffled," Robin told Jennifer. "I started to read and research the power of positive prayer and came upon dozens of medical studies that proved it's an effective medicine."

Robin emphasized that she was not talking about faith healing or New Age hocus-pocus.

"I got my information from scientific studies conducted at Duke University and other top schools," she said. "I felt the evidence was strong that patients make remarkable progress when they know there are people pulling for them in a united way."

Robin suggested a prayer chain.

Jennifer said it couldn't hurt.

"I just kind of immediately clicked with her," Jennifer said. "She was a complete stranger who was eager to do something to help us—something that was meaningful and positive."

But Robin said she would not proceed with the idea unless Jarrett approved.

Jennifer put Jarrett on the phone, and Robin explained what she had in mind.

"Absolutely, I want it," Jarrett said, emphatically. "It's not my time to go."

And with that blessing, Robin hung up and began crafting the words to a prayer solely for a boy she had never met.

"I didn't want to set Jarrett up for unrealistic results," Jennifer said. "We were rational about his condition. But so many people would come up to me and say, 'We're concerned about Jarrett. What can we do to help?' I never knew what to say before. Now, I thought, I could hand them this prayer and ask them to join our chain."

Robin didn't pretend that she could write words that would make Jarrett well.

"What I could do was stir up a lot of love around him," she said. "Everybody has this ability, but not everyone is a writer. Therefore, my words make a lot of sense to those who don't know what to say to God."

Robin wrote a prayer that may seem too generic to some people. But that was on purpose. She wanted it to be distributed to Christians, Jews, Muslims, and Buddhists. She asked that the readers adapt the wording to match their normal prayer practices.

"I wanted people to personalize it," she said. "Put it in Christ's name, if that's whom you say your prayers to." Robin, who is Jewish, didn't even know the Mynears were Roman Catholics. She didn't ask. It didn't matter.

"The more faiths, the better," Robin said. "God seems to like it when we put aside our differences."

The prayer was all positive. It didn't contain negative language such as "Please don't let Jarrett die." It was a thank you for sustaining him through the tough times:

> *Source of Life,*
> *We have come together as one heart, one voice,*
> *To ask Your blessing on Jarrett Mynear.*
> *Take our love and deliver it to him now.*
> *Use it for his highest good.*
> *May what we offer of ourselves comfort and soothe him.*

Let his body receive the positive energy we offer,
Using it to strengthen the organs, muscles, bones, nerves, and tissues
that sustain life.
Be with him now, as You are with us, in life.
Bless Jarrett and his family with Your grace.
Thank You, thank You for the peace that embraces us in this effort.
May all be well. May all be free.
Amen.

Jennifer e-mailed the prayer to all of her friends and relatives and asked them to pass it on. Robin did the same. The message requested that everyone say the prayer at 9 P.M., Eastern Standard Time, if possible. If not, they should say it whenever it was convenient.

"Nine o'clock was the about the time Jarrett was going to bed each night," Robin said. "I felt it would be good for him to slip into sleep while people were sending out thousands of beams of love."

The Internet can spread a message like wildlife. Consider how quickly a virus can infect computers around the world. And anyone who goes online knows how common it is to see the same jokes, chain letters, and hoaxes pop up in their e-mail time and time again.

The prayer chain spread the same way. In a matter of days, Jennifer began to receive e-mail from all over North America, as well as Europe and the Middle East. Rosie O'Donnell posted the prayer on her website, after giving her third on-air update on Jarrett's condition.

"I got letters from missionaries in Africa who said they were saying the prayer," Jennifer said. "It was incredible to think each evening people all over the world were praying for him. Complete strangers would come up to me in stores and tell me they were saying the prayer.

"I was a little embarrassed at first. I thought people might think we were expecting too much. But even months later, I never had one negative comment about it."

Much of Jarrett's faith was shaped by his friendship with Maurice Adkins, the man who fitted him with each artificial leg he had over the years.

Maurice owned a home in his native Pike County, three hours from Lexington. He and his wife spent every weekend there, and they invited Jarrett to visit at least twice a year.

Jarrett loved that mountain getaway, near hiking trails and fishing holes. Maurice would let Jarrett shoot a pistol at targets, and he would take him to go-cart tracks and knife shows.

"Jennifer told me I was going to turn her son into a redneck," Maurice laughed. "But the visits were good for both of us. It kept me young and kept him from thinking so much about his cancer."

Maurice was on a diving team in his youth, and during one visit, when Jarrett was eight, the boy was determined to get his pal back on the board.

"I hadn't done a front flip in twenty-five years," Maurice remembered. "Jarrett wanted me to show him how it was done. I told him I was too old and out of shape, but he wouldn't let me off the hook that easily."

"C'mon," Jarrett coaxed. "If you do one, I'll do one."

After much goading, Maurice stepped up on the diving board and looked out over the water in his backyard pool. He had a second thought . . . then a third thought . . . and started to step back down. But then he spied Jarrett, sitting on the edge of the pool with catheters in his chest, wide-eyed with anticipation.

And in an instant, Maurice extended his arms in front of him and flipped into the pool, slicing the water like a hot knife through butter.

When he surfaced, Jarrett was standing there cheering.

Then the boy made his way to the diving board.

"He must've gone off that board ten times in a row," Maurice said. "I don't think he ever did completely flip over, but he swears he did."

What a sight it must have been—a grandfatherly figure and a tiny eight-year-old, both laughing and splashing like crazy in the pool, challenging each other to "do it again." And neither one of them had a right leg. Some people might have questioned whether they had their right minds.

Maurice restored antique cars. His pride and joy was a cherry red 1934 Plymouth coupe.

"It's really souped up," Maurice said.

Jarrett loved to go riding in the old car, sitting on a pillow so he could see over the dashboard and maybe so people in the other cars could see him they passed.

Both driver and passenger felt pretty cool when they were "cruising."

"Once when I was taking him home, Jarrett said to me, 'I thought you said this was a hot rod. Why are you going so slowly?'" Maurice said.

"So, I hit the pedal to the floor and the force pinned him back in the seat. His mother would've killed me if she had known.

"He straightened up and had a big smile on his face. He said, 'Do it again.' So, I did, and we both laughed like hyenas. My wife stopped going out with us. She said we acted too silly and made too much noise. We embarrassed her!"

It was that spirit that inspired Maurice and, like Robin Silverman, he wanted to surround his friend with the positive power of prayer.

Maurice attended a little country church. He described it as "old-time Methodist."

He had added Jarrett's name to the church's prayer list right after he met him as a toddler.

"The congregation prayed for him every week for years, even though it hadn't met him," Maurice said. "I kept telling the members how special he was, and not a week went by when I didn't give them an update on his condition."

Finally, in his eighth year, Jarrett went to church with Maurice on one of his visits to Pike County. He wanted to meet the people who had been praying for him, and the congregation was happy to put a face with the name it had been lifting to the Lord.

The country preacher asked Jarrett if he would like to say a few words—a question to which Jarrett never answered "no."

Jarrett walked to the front of the sanctuary and thanked the churchgoers for their support.

"I know you've been praying for me, and that means a lot," Jarrett said. "Maurice told me that God put him and me together for a reason, and it's been great. Maurice always puts me in a good mood. When I'm feeling down, I can call him and he makes me feel better. I think it's important to have good friends, and he's been my best friend. And even though most of you don't know me, I know about you. You're all my friends, too."

Jarrett's sincerity stirred the congregation.

"There wasn't a dry eye in the house," Maurice said. "The sermon was good that day, but nothing was as uplifting as Jarrett's speech."

When the service was over, Maurice and Jarrett walked toward the car.

"Did you feel that?" Jarrett asked his host.

"Feel what?" Maurice asked back.

"God was in there," Jarrett said.

The observation caused Maurice to pause.

"Yes, He was Jarrett. And now He's out here. He's going with you wherever you go."

In 1999, Maurice had open-heart surgery. There were complications, and the operation left him weak and somewhat depressed. In fact, doctors told him there was a chance he would not live much longer.

Jarrett didn't know how serious it was. Maurice hadn't wanted to worry him.

"The first night after coming home from the hospital, I felt sad and sorry for myself," Maurice recalled. "The phone rang at 10 o'clock that night, just as I was getting ready for bed. There was Jarrett's happy voice on the other end saying, 'Hey buddy, I thought you might need a little cheering up!'"

Maurice's mood changed instantly.

"I thought, 'Here's this kid who's been through so much, and he's thinking about me.' I never asked God for another day after that. I realized how blessed I was. And it was Jarrett who opened my eyes."

In late 2000, as Jarrett struggled through his toughest time yet, the pair sat at a table in a pizza parlor, waiting for a pepperoni pie with extra cheese.

Maurice knew how bad things were. He had seen the blisters in Jarrett's throat and had heard from the boy's mother about the numerous tumors that had shown up on the most recent x-rays.

"You're not feeling too well, are you?" he asked Jarrett.

The boy reached his small hands across the table and took Maurice's hands. The tears began to flow.

"They think I'm gonna die," Jarrett confided.

"What do you think?"

"I don't think they're right," Jarrett said. "I can't go yet. I have too much to do."

"Then that's the way you handle it," Maurice instructed. "Keep doing all you need to do. God won't let you leave here with unfinished business."

"That's what I think too," Jarrett said. "I'm still perfecting my front flip."

41

Penny War

Just after Christmas, the principal at West Jessamine Middle School issued a challenge to the student body. He told the students if they could raise $3,000 to help pay for Jarrett's medical expenses, he would shave his head. And better still, the kids who raised the most money could do the shearing.

And The Penny War was on.

Several of the teachers had talked with Glen Teater, the principal, about doing something to help Jarrett's entire family. The Mynears really didn't need any more toys for the cart right then, but the bills had to be mounting. The teachers said the students seemed to be really down about the news that Jarrett was doing so poorly. Many of them had asked how they could "make it better."

"When the teachers came to me with the idea, I was reluctant at first," Jennifer said. "We were so much more fortunate than many of the families, and we weren't comfortable having them collect money for our own benefit."

But the teachers and staffers knew insurance didn't cover all of Jarrett's expenses. The Mynears spent more than $10,000 a year out of their own pockets. That had added up to more than $100,000 over the years. The school staff insisted that a collection drive would be good for the students.

Doug and Jennifer gave their permission for The Penny War, on one condition. They said they would put the money in the bank and let it draw interest. They would use some for traveling expenses and medical bills, but they also wanted to find a way to make it benefit the school. Perhaps down the road, it would need library books or a computer or some other piece of equipment. Months later, the Mynears used some of the proceeds to fly

Jarrett's friend Greg Siegman in from Chicago to conduct assemblies about diversity and racial harmony at several schools in the county.

The rules of a penny war are difficult to explain. The kids seemed to comprehend it better than the adults did.

Basically, a jar was placed in each homeroom, and kids would deposit their change there. A penny counted as one point. But the student could also go into other rooms and make deposits. Coins other than pennies resulted in negative points for that room. For example, if a jar had twenty-five pennies in it, that meant twenty-five points. But if a student dropped in a dime, ten points were subtracted. So, the jar would contain thirty-five cents, but be worth just fifteen points.

It was a way to "slam" your competition while still causing the pot to grow. The competition grew fierce, with teachers getting involved too. Jars that one day looked completely copper-colored would show a top layer of silver the next day.

"Kids literally brought in buckets full of change," Jennifer said, laughing. "They were forcing their family members to cough it up."

Once again, it was an incredible show of school support and proof that giving can be as much fun as receiving.

At the end of January, Mr. Teater called an assembly to announce the result of "the war."

"Before I do this," he said, "I want us to welcome back our friend Jarrett Mynear."

Jarrett walked into the gym for the first time since mid-November. Every student rose and applauded. The cheers and whistles rang around the hollow room. Jennifer stood along a wall and wiped tears from her eyes.

Then Mr. Teater talked to the students about the sense of community that had developed over the past few weeks and reminded them again about what it means to be charitable.

The gym broke out into the school chant: "West is best . . . West is best … West is best."

Mr. Teater let it continue for a couple of minutes, and then quieted the crowd with a wave of his arms.

"I guess you're wondering how much money we raised," he said. "Remember, I'm not going to shave my head unless it's $3,000."

The students fidgeted in the bleachers and smiled devilish grins. They were sure they had met the goal.

"Well, here's the total," Teater said, building suspense as he fumbled to unfold a sheet of paper.

"Let's see . . . it looks like . . . let me be sure . . . yeah . . . $6,500!"

The room echoed with laughter and applause. The take more than doubled the goal.

"Before I lose my hair, I want anybody in this room who had anything at all to do with this to stand and be recognized, even if you gave just one penny."

Everyone stood, including teachers, cooks, janitors, and office aides.

Love isn't something you can hold in your hand, but it is something you can feel. Jarrett felt it multiplied seven hundred and fifty times as he looked at all those people on their feet. He later told his mom that assembly meant more to him than any award he had ever received.

Two teachers brought a tarpaulin out to cover the gym floor, and they turned a bucket upside down as a seat for Mr. Teater.

The five kids who had raised the most money were called up to help with the honors. Each one took a swipe with the electric clippers as the student body roared its approval and Mr. Teater's locks hit the floor.

Then they handed the clippers to Jarrett, who delighted in cutting a stripe from his principal's crown to his forehead.

Then, he stopped and reached into a bag at his side. Jarrett pulled out a child-sized wig.

"I thought you might want to wear this," Jarrett said, handing it to Mr. Teater. "I never really used it."

It was an ugly wig, Jennifer admits—one she had purchased years before thinking Jarrett might be self-conscious about his baldness. That was an unfounded worry. The wig became more of a joke. It looked like a dead squirrel. Mr. Teater was welcome to it.

The principal was scheduled to go with a Kentucky delegation to

Washington later that week. He would attend the inauguration of President George W. Bush.

"It will be cold in Washington," Jarrett said. "This wig will keep you warm."

Jennifer got a mental image of Mr. Teater meeting the President with the pathetic hairpiece balanced on top of his shiny pate. She laughed out loud.

A science teacher, Donny Loughry, took a straight razor and shaving cream and finished the job, leaving the principal with a sleek chrome dome.

Another teacher, whose hobby was sewing, came forward with two red and white fleece hats she had made. They had earflaps like Elmer Fudd would wear in a Looney Tunes cartoon. Jarrett and Mr. Teater both left the school that day sporting the funky headgear. To be truthful, Jarrett still felt miserable, but the assembly had been a great morale booster.

As the buses pulled away, a custodian swept up the stray salt and pepper locks on the gym floor. The principal may have given up his hair, but everyone in the school had shown their roots—strands of compassion that were buried deep and would continue to grow.

By mid-March, the scans showed the tumors were shrinking. Jennifer was certain The Penny War and the prayer chain had made a difference.

Robin Silverman, the prayer chain's author, got to know Jarrett and his family better through the effort, and she said the experience changed her life.

"Jarrett seemed to know a secret about life that the rest of us just don't know," she said. "In his soul agreement, I believe he was told to come down here from Heaven and teach us all about love."

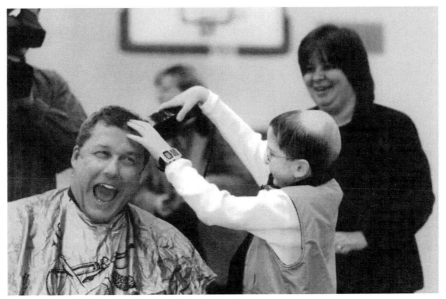

Jarrett shaves Principal Glen Teater's head as
curriculum coordinator Margie Maloney looks on

(Staff photo/ Lexington Herald-Leader)

42

Reflection

As Jennifer stood in the warehouse on a warm spring day, facing boxes stacked to the ceiling, she thought about the big job she had ahead of her. She had an inventory list in one hand and a yellow highlighter in the other. She needed to see if everything Toys "R" Us shipped had actually made it to Lexington. This was the booty from a fourth appearance on *The Rosie O'Donnell Show* in which the toy company had pledged to send another $10,000 worth of donations.

Jennifer would have to restack the boxes, putting toys for infants along one wall and separating those best suited for older boys and girls along another wall. It was incredible to see what the company had sent: building blocks, baby rattles, Barbie dolls, dress-up clothes for girls and cowboy hats for boys, Play-Doh molds, wood burning sets, model airplanes, Nerf basketballs and hoops, yo-yos, compact discs, music boxes, backpacks, plastic horses, and rubber snakes. Soon, Terry Hagan of The Dream Factory would be there to help move boxes, and warehouse workers would bring in pallets and forklifts to relocate the stacks away from the entrance.

But as she stood there waiting for the helping hands, in the musty space with sunlight streaming through skylights and cobwebs glistening in the rafters, it seemed as if she were facing a giant beast made of cardboard and packing tape.

"When The Joy Cart started, none of us had any idea what we were getting ourselves into," she said later. The pet project had turned into a monster, albeit a friendly one. When it needed to be fed, donors always came through. The cart never went hungry.

There, in the warehouse in an isolated section of the city, was the part of The Joy Cart no one ever saw—the part that was hard work. In a back room, way beyond rows of business records and millions of documents that were stored there, was the toy storage room. It had once been a break room for employees of a large bakery that had abandoned the warehouse nearly a decade earlier. Jarrett had never seen this part of his operation. He couldn't come here because of allergies to dust and mold.

This was not just a Toys "R" Us mountain. Other boxes contained toys collected by school groups, churches, and civic clubs, and donations from stores that had cleared shelves as they went out of business. In some ways, the room was like a museum. Many of the toys were discontinued items—things you could not buy any longer. And every week, like clockwork, Jennifer came here to pick and choose items to load into the family van. The toys would go from here to the hospital to be loaded onto carts for the next run.

"It amazed me every time I went there to see how much people had donated," Jennifer said. "If I ever started to gripe about having so many boxes to climb over, I'd stop and remind myself that this was an outpouring of love from a lot of people who care about Jarrett and believe in him."

The response had quite possibly given Jarrett the will to live during some tough times. It is what put the joy in The Joy Cart.

This was a good place to think.

Just six hours after Jarrett had been diagnosed with cancer for the first time, when he was two-and-a-half years old, a retired priest told Jennifer "to look for the good in this." It had made her angry.

"It's not what I wanted to hear," she said. "I wanted to throw him out of the hospital when he said that."

But now, when she wanted to look for the good in Jarrett's situation, she could see it in this stuffy warehouse.

"We have been blessed because so many people have reached out to us," she said, "not only by giving toys, but also giving of their time. They've helped us clean the house, they've brought us meals, provided babysitting, and prayed for us every night.

"We'd get bogged down thinking how we could pay everybody back, and then just realized it would never be possible. When you can't pay back, you pay it forward and just do something nice for someone else."

That was the whole concept of The Joy Cart in a nutshell.

Jennifer thought about all the places they had been, all the people they had met, all the doors that had opened because of Jarrett's cancer.

Their son lived a compressed life, doing more in his first twelve years than most people could hope to do in a lifetime.

"We really are better people because of what has happened," Jennifer said.

That doesn't mean she would go back and do it all over again, given the chance to change things.

"It's absurd to think we're dancing in the streets saying cancer's been wonderful for us," she said. "No one would choose this."

Jarrett had been an inspiration to so many that Jennifer believed sometimes people thought he was superhuman.

"There were a couple of times when he had to unload his emotions. We learned early on not to waste too much energy dwelling on things we couldn't change. We didn't want him to spend time asking 'Why me?' and go on about how unfair it was. But we had to let him validate his feelings."

Only once did she really see Jarrett snap. It was in private at their home.

"He said, 'I'm sick of being little bitty, having to crane my neck every time I look at somebody. I'm sick of worrying about the port-o-cath in my side and at people expecting me to be happy all the time. And I wish the girls would look at me as someone they might want to go out with someday and not just as everybody's little buddy.'"

Jennifer let him vent.

"I thought, at least that once, it was healthy. It's normal to feel that way."

Jennifer knew how tough it was for her to suck it up and be tough sometimes. She couldn't imagine what it was like for a twelve-year-old boy.

"Sometimes I'd be so tired I couldn't think straight," she said. "Many times I'd tell Doug to just get the car and drive us to a restaurant because I couldn't focus enough to put something on the stove. Jarrett's ability to keep it together always amazed me."

As she continued sifting through the donations, Jennifer thought how much better it was to be there than in the pediatric clinic, where she had spent a large portion of her life waiting for her son to go through his chemotherapy.

"It was just emotionally draining to sit there," she said. "All of the children there are in the same condition as Jarrett or worse. It's a room full of parents watching their kids get infused with poisons. You're just immersed in the world of cancer.

"I've formed countless friendships with the other mothers who come there, and I've watched many of them bury their children. I witnessed a six-year-old girl screaming at the top of her lungs, 'Just let me die!' That's why it's hard to accept it when well-meaning people say 'Look for the good in this.'"

She has also watched marriages break apart, as mothers had to quit their jobs.

"The wives say to their husbands, 'You don't know what it's like to spend all day at the clinic,' and the husbands say, 'Well, you don't know it's like to be at work all day wondering what's happening but not being able to leave because someone has to bring home a paycheck.'"

She and Doug had had similar conversations.

But again, she looked at the donations stacked in front of her and thought how, despite all the work, Jarrett's idea had been their salvation. It gave him, and all of them, a reason to keep going.

"During the weeks when I couldn't run the cart and I left it in the hands of volunteers, I'd find myself wondering which kids had been at the hospital that week and how they were doing. And when Jarrett couldn't go, he'd ask me who was there. I'd see him get excited when he spied certain toys in the back of the van. He'd say, 'So-and-so's there. He's gonna love that.'"

And even though she was too young to go on the patient floors at the children's hospital, Claire took ownership in The Joy Cart as well. She made suggestions about what toys to take to the little girls and always helped load the van.

"It was her way of being able to help out," Jennifer said.

As she got older, Jarrett worried that Claire might be jealous of all the attention he received. But, somewhat surprisingly, her parents marveled at the way she handled Jarrett's fame.

She refused to be overlooked. For one thing, she was bigger than Jarrett. At age nine, her 5'2" height was a full foot taller than her brother's twelve-year-old frame. She weighed 30 pounds more.

"When a stranger ignored her, it probably wasn't on purpose," Jennifer said. "They probably didn't even know Jarrett had a little sister."

Time and time again, Doug and Jennifer watched Claire come up and introduce herself to someone who was talking to Jarrett.

"She'd stick out her hand and proudly say, 'I'm Claire. I'm his sister and I gave him my bone marrow.'"

It always made them smile.

When Jarrett had speeches and other public appearances, Claire often stayed home, simply because she didn't want to go.

"She had had more than her fill of banquets and boring speeches," Jennifer said. "We didn't want people to think we were leaving her behind. For her, it was a treat to get a night at home with her own babysitter. Then she was the center of attention in her own domain."

Children with ADHD need as much predictability as possible, and with the Mynears' situation, nothing was predictable.

"When Claire first went to school, she couldn't handle it if someone else came to pick her up after school, even someone she knew and loved," Jennifer said. "If I wasn't there, she'd immediately worry that something was wrong with Jarrett."

So Jennifer made it a point to be in the school's parking lot each day, as often as possible, even when that meant a half-hour drive from the hospital to the school to home and back to the hospital.

"But the longer she was in school and socializing with other people, the more she matured," Jennifer said. "She became better able to handle a lack of predictability."

The patients at the hospital also had trouble dealing with a break from the routine. One week, about four months after The Joy Cart began, there was just no one available to take it on its regular Tuesday night run—the only time that had ever happened.

A young cancer patient named Stanley stayed awake until 2 A.M. He just knew that Jarrett would be coming. The boy's mother told him Jarrett is not like Santa Claus. He doesn't come in the middle of the night. But Stanley insisted that Jarrett wouldn't forget him.

Finally, the nurses found an unopened toy they had stashed away in the playroom and gave it to him, telling him it was from Jarrett.

Stanley fell asleep, clutching a Matchbox car in his hand.

Jennifer remembered the story and laughed out loud.

That was the good in all this.

43

Sequel

Melinda Morrison knew a lot of business and media leaders in Seattle, and the more she thought about it, the more she knew it was the right place for Jarrett's Joy Cart II. He had spent so much time in the city, it was where he had his stem cell transplants, and there was a lot about the Northwest that Jarrett loved.

So right after the segment aired on Oprah, she began working behind the scenes in a much more proactive way than the Mynears knew.

Melinda showed the videotape of the Oprah segment and several press clippings to the administrators at the Seattle Children's Hospital. They liked the idea.

That hospital had recently teamed with The Hutch. Children who came from all over the world for bone marrow and stem cells transplants stayed there. It had more than 600 beds—twelve times more than the children's hospital in Kentucky.

Melinda contacted other people the Mynears knew there, including Jarrett's former teacher, Susan Sever, and Paul Gordon, the young documentary producer he had met at the Prudential Spirit of Community awards. They promised to help.

And she called on Howard Lincoln, the CEO of the Seattle Mariners. He told Melinda whenever she was ready, the organization would set up a royal welcome for Jarrett by providing his family with a hotel room and hosting a reception for them at the ballpark.

Melinda took a leave of absence from *The Oprah Winfrey Show*.

"I e-mailed her (Oprah) and told her I was following the advice she always preaches—that you should follow your passion," Melinda said.

She worked feverishly to collect toys and line up sponsors, and when she had her ducks in a row, Melinda called Jennifer.

"I need you to be in Seattle the first week in April," she said over the phone, wanting Jarrett to be at the Mariner's season opener.

"Well, I'm not sure we can make it," Jennifer said. "Everything is touch and go with Jarrett right now. He may not be able to travel."

But Melinda made Jennifer promise to try to make the trip if at all possible. She understood about the uncertainty of Jarrett's health. All she was asking was that she and Doug clear their work schedules and be on standby, in the event Jarrett was having a good week.

"I bought the plane tickets," Melinda said. "I just put them on my credit card. I didn't care. I'd figure out how to pay for them later."

When his parents told Jarrett about the planned rollout of a second Joy Cart in Seattle, he perked up. It was what he had hoped for.

"I didn't do this to become famous," he said. "But I would like to see it expand beyond Kentucky. I want to be there for the ribbon cutting."

The family had plane tickets for Saturday, March 31st. But the night before, Jarrett came down with a fever. A quick trip to the doctor resulted in a night in the hospital. Based on past experience, the family wasn't about to fly while Jarrett was running a temperature.

But by Monday, Jarrett seemed as spunky as ever. His parents knew he was eager to go to Seattle. And, even though they seldom allowed themselves to think that way, they realized his days might be numbered.

"We wanted him to see his good works being multiplied," Jennifer said. "He had been so sick and so weak since November, we thought we'd better take this window of opportunity. This may be the best he'd ever feel again."

Jennifer called Melinda and told her they would come, because she had a strong feeling this would be the family's last vacation as a foursome.

That thought broke Melinda's heart.

So, Doug, Jennifer, Claire, and Jarrett got reissued tickets and flew to Seattle on April 2, 2001. Melinda met them at the airport.

"I wasn't prepared to see Jarrett that way," she said. "He was really weak, and his dad carried him. I didn't know if I could handle it."

A limo whisked the family to the Westin Hotel, compliments of the Mariners.

When they opened the door to their room, it was the most beautiful suite they had ever stayed in. It had two bedrooms with separate space for the kids. It was clear the Mariners didn't do anything halfway.

The next afternoon, the family went to Safeco Field and got the grand tour.

During the practice session, almost every player came over to shake Jarrett's hand and pose for pictures with him. It was clear they had been briefed on who their special guest was and what he had accomplished.

"Jarrett rallied," Melinda observed. "He seemed so much stronger than he had the day before. He was running on adrenaline and sheer willpower."

Jarrett asked infielder Mark McLemore to sign a baseball. McLemore pulled a ball out of his own pocket and said, "You don't need my autograph, I need yours. I saw you on Oprah."

"They were all the nicest bunch of guys," Jennifer said. "It was incredible. They went out on the field to do stretches, and they made sure Jarrett did them too."

When the players left the field to go to the locker rooms, Doug and Jarrett were invited in, too. They just hung out in the clubhouse a while, taking in the entire pre-game atmosphere.

The family had dinner in the president's suite, enjoying the all-they-could eat buffet. It sure beat stadium hot dogs.

About fifteen minutes before the Mariners were about to meet the Oakland Athletics on that cold night, a Mariners staffer escorted the family back down to the edge of the field. The public address system blared as the announcer told the crowd about that night's ceremonial first pitch.

Jarrett's name flashed on the scoreboard in huge white lights, and the fans in the stands watched a short video clip that explained The Joy Cart. Melinda had supplied some of her video from the Oprah show. The Mariners production department had also dropped in some last-minute scenes from Jarrett's pre-game visits with the players.

"Chills ran up my spine as I looked up at that scoreboard and all those people," Jennifer said. "Here we were more than two thousand miles from home, and our son was the center of attention. To see all of his work coming to fruition in another city was almost unbelievable."

Melinda also felt the electricity. Even months later, she couldn't talk about it without crying.

"It was the highlight of my life so far," she said.

When the clip ended, the Mariner's mascot, a large costumed moose, led Jarrett to a spot just in front of the pitcher's mound.

Forty-five thousand fans stood and cheered.

"I thought, 'O.K., I've done what I wanted to do,'" Melinda said. ""I can't cure him, but this is the best I can do.'"

Jarrett wound up and let the ball fly right across home plate. The crowd responded with applause that soared through the chilly night air.

The moose presented Jarrett with two large shopping bags full of Mariner's souvenirs—t-shirts, caps, teddy bears, and pennants that he could use to help stock the newest Joy Cart.

A member of the team's organization walked the family back to the owner's suite where they spent the evening with Melinda and several other people who had made the night possible, including owner Howard Lincoln and executives from Boeing.

The stadium may have been full of renowned athletes and executives, but Jarrett was treated like the MVP.

Melinda relished watching Jarrett as he enjoyed every minute of the evening.

"He was chatting with the bartender and the servers in the presidential suite as if to say, 'This is the way it's supposed to be,'" she said, laughing.

As the evening wore on, Jennifer decided it was time to go. It was just the seventh inning, but another big day was ahead. It was the only time Melinda had seen Jarrett get testy.

"I'm not ready to go," Jarrett protested.

"Ready or not, it's time," Jennifer responded.

"I get an allowance. You go on. I'll use my own money to get a taxi," Jarrett said.

"No, you'll go with us now," Jennifer said.

"Mom, I have cancer. Let me stay," he replied, trying to play the sympathy card.

"Cancer or not, you're going," his mother said, winning the battle.

Melinda knew she probably shouldn't delight in witnessing the argument. But it was the payoff to all of her planning. It meant Jarrett was having a great time.

The next day, with the excitement of the game not yet worn off, Jarrett and his family went to the Seattle Children's Hospital.

They walked into the playroom, and the scene took them back two years. It was much like the news conference in Kentucky in 1999 when they had the inaugural run of Jarrett's Joy Cart. Just like then, the room was full of television cameras, reporters, and still photographers. Hospital administrators, doctors, and nurses lined the walls.

One of the first people Doug and Jennifer spied was John Hayes, the volunteer from The Hutch who had arranged the troll skit and so many other surprises for Jarrett. It had been five years since they had seen each other. Walt Disney was right. It's a small world after all.

"I thought it was great for all these people he had known to see he had done this amazing thing," Melinda said.

Once again, Jarrett's parents stood back and watched in amazement as their son talked to the media about the idea behind The Joy Cart—the simple yet profound message he had repeated so many times.

"This is about giving kids something to look forward to," Jarrett said again, with as much conviction as the first time he uttered the phrase.

A hospital cart sat in front of the room loaded down with stuffed animals, puzzles, books, and trinkets. The sign on the front of it said "**JARRETT'S SEATTLE JOY CART.**" A red ribbon draped across the front.

Melinda handed Jarrett a pair of scissors, and he bent down on his artificial right knee and snipped the ribbon in two.

Cameras flashed, and two pre-selected children came in for the photo op, picking the first two toys off the cart.

They turned and smiled.

The joy had spread.

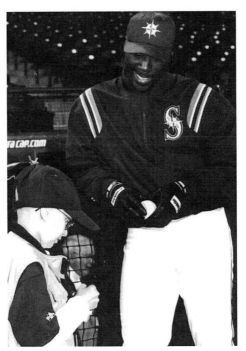

Jarrett autographs a baseball for
Mark McLemore of The Seattle Mariners

(Photo/Gerry Morrison)

44
Some Good Days

Jarrett beat the odds so many times that there was nothing predictable about him. He was proof that a positive attitude could be better than any medicine.

"He really does care about other people, and he's found the perfect way to communicate that," Dr. Moscow said when he knew the end was near. "He has found the perfect way to harness his natural interest in other patients."

"So many people care very deeply about him," the doctor said. "Eventually, we'll run out of tricks. We'll reach into our bag, and there will be nothing left. Jarrett knows that. That's why it's so important that he makes every day of his life special."

In the final months, there were still special days.

Jarrett had another great idea that he and his mother worked on throughout the fall. They decided that in December they would take two weeks and run The Joy Cart in reverse. Instead of coming to their bedsides, volunteers would escort the young patients to a room set up like a store. And instead of picking a toy for themselves, the children would be allowed to "shop" for their parents, siblings, and other family members. It was a way to let the patients share in the joy of giving.

Jennifer said Jarrett literally ran the operation from his hospital bed. He wrote down ideas for gift items and made signs for "Jarrett's Joy Cart Holiday Store." He told anyone who came to visit him what he had in mind, hoping they would donate. Of course, most of them did. Jennifer made several trips to department stores, knowing they would need hundreds of gifts to make this effort a success.

In early December, a multi-purpose room at the hospital was converted into a store where all of the merchandise was free. Tables were set up, filled with things an adult might like such as perfume, tools, gloves, candles, boxes of chocolate, and coffee mugs.

On a Joy Cart Tuesday night, Jarrett was filled with excitement as his dad wheeled him into the room. He donned a Santa hat and took up a position near the door. Volunteers brought a few children at a time into the store. Many patients clutched a shopping list as Jarrett greeted them and told them to have fun.

He loved watching the kids pick out gifts, and it was a long process for some of them. They wanted to see all of their options. Many of them, who had been in hospitals so much of their lives, had never had a chance to give a gift that they had chosen themselves to their mom, dad, or sibling.

"No one seemed to mind that they weren't getting a toy for themselves that week," Jennifer said. "The kids were excited about the idea of surprising their loved ones with Christmas gifts. Some of them were downright giddy."

Volunteers wrapped the gifts, and Jarrett helped the patients make tags. Jarrett had been referred to as "Santa Claus" many times since he started The Joy Cart. The nickname was never more fitting than on the night he opened the holiday store. From now on, I will always imagine Santa as a small boy with a bald spot on his head and an artificial leg.

On December 17, 2001, the Olympic flame came through central Kentucky. More than 11,500 torchbearers would carry the flame as it made its way across the country to the Winter Games in Salt Lake City. The carriers were chosen from 210,000 nominees, each with a personal story worthy of recognition. Jarrett had been nominated by numerous people, including Mark Maloney, a sportswriter for the *Lexington Herald-Leader*.

Mark, who had donated a kidney to a friend, was selected to run with the torch on a street near the state capitol in Frankfort.

"It was a big honor for me," he said, recalling how drivers stopped their cars to honk as he passed them. "The Olympic flame makes everyone smile."

But Mark knew he was not the big celebrity torchbearer of the day. That would be Jarrett. So he rushed back to Lexington, took a quick shower at the newspaper office, and grabbed a spot on the sidewalk to wait for Jarrett to pass. Mark's wife, Margie, who was Jarrett's homebound teacher and the assistant principal at West Jessamine Middle School, had tipped him off that busloads of students and cheerleaders would be lining the three blocks assigned to Jarrett.

No one waiting for Jarrett that day could have known how miserable he felt. His family had just found out days before that there were four more tumors in his brain.

"His right arm went numb the night before the relay," Doug said. "He had no real control or strength in that arm. The latest round of chemotherapy was taking its toll, but he wasn't about to back out of carrying the torch."

Doug and Jarrett got on a shuttle bus at the edge of Main Street and were dropped off at the designated handoff spot.

After a few minutes, the flame came into view, being carried by a reporter from the *St. Louis Post-Dispatch*. Cynthia Billhartz later wrote that she was a last-minute fill-in. She was on the bus to write a story about the relay, not to run it.

"Fortunately, no one asked me why I was running the torch," she wrote. She said she didn't feel she belonged in the company of the other torchbearers, but her discomfort turned into curiosity and she realized it would give her a unique firsthand perspective for her article.

A few people waved and applauded as the reporter ran with the flame, but when she rounded the last corner, the air was filled with thunderous cheers. She was amazed at how many people lined the next street on the relay route— all there to see tiny Jarrett.

She touched her torch to his, passing the flame, and watched as he turned and walked down the street. He took it slowly, finding the strength to keep the three-pound torch at shoulder level. The cheers and applause rolled in waves as Jarrett progressed.

"Way to go, Jarrett, way to go," his classmates chanted. Jennifer wiped tears from her cheeks as she and Doug followed a few steps behind. They knew how bad things were, but somehow, their son was still able to put on his best face, glowing like the flame in his hands.

"I just remember how big his smile was," said Mark Maloney. "It was cool for me to carry the flame, but the highlight of my day was seeing Jarrett carry it. You could just feel love in the crowd."

"As a sportswriter, I've interviewed a lot of people with big names, such as LeBron James or Randall Cobb. But my hero is Jarrett."

After walking for three blocks, Jarrett handed off the flame to Collier Mills, a 6' 8" basketball player from Transylvania University. "Oh, great! I gotta light a tall guy," joked the boy, who was 4' 1."

But to those who knew him best, Jarrett seemed like a giant that day.

In early 2002, Jarrett's aunt, Margaret Wagner, decided if her nephew's idea could spread to the West Coast, then it should also expand into Kentucky's largest city. She arranged to have Jarrett go with her to meet with members of the Kosair Children's Hospital Foundation in Louisville. Jarrett did most of the talking.

"They were so impressed with him and The Joy Cart that they got on board immediately," Margaret said. She had not expected to get the green light so quickly.

It didn't surprise Guy Jones, the loyal volunteer who helped with the Lexington operation. He said the cart has always seemed to have an invisible push behind it.

"You and I probably wouldn't make it past the door," Guy said. "If not for Jarrett walking in those board rooms and asking for permission, the idea would've never gotten off the ground. How could you say 'no' to him?"

In June, Jarrett once again got to take scissors in hand and cut the ribbon on a Joy Cart— his third.

"He was in a wheelchair and not feeling very well that day," Margaret recalled. "But he insisted on going into a couple of the patient rooms and handing out the first toys."

He never told anyone he was feeling bad. All those kids with cancer saw was a survivor who told them things were going to get better.

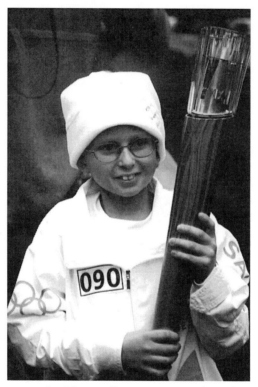

Jarrett carries the Olympic flame as it passes through Lexington on the way to Salt Lake City, December 17, 2001

45

Joy in the Mourning

By August 2002, Jarrett's family knew the doctors had run out of options. The bag of tricks was about to come up empty. You never want to allow yourself to think all hope is gone, but there comes a time when you have to face the inevitable. You have to prepare for the day you have dreaded for years. Jarrett's body grew weaker, and the tumors grew larger as his kidneys and liver began to shut down.

"Jarrett and I had a few conversations about death and him leaving," his mother said. "But he did not want to say a lot of goodbyes. He certainly didn't want to talk to counselors about death, although he acknowledged it."

In the final weeks, the hospital assigned a young social worker to Jarrett. Rick McClung came to the house almost daily, hoping he could help Jarrett deal with any depression or concerns he may have. But any time Rick tried to get into a deep discussion, Jarrett changed the subject. He just wanted Rick to be his video game partner.

"Rick took me aside one day when he was at the house and said, 'I don't think I'm doing any good here,'" Jennifer said. "He was bothered that Jarrett wouldn't open up about his feelings.

"I told him he was doing more good than he'd ever know," she said. "Jarrett loved Rick and looked forward to his visits. Playing games with him was the best therapy possible."

On the last day of September, a Monday, Jennifer carried Jarrett from his bedroom to their downstairs living room and propped him up with some pillows on the sofa. As she was heading to the kitchen for a cup of coffee, Jarrett said, "I need you to call Rick."

The time had come when Jarrett was ready for a serious talk.

Rick came right over. Jennifer stayed in the kitchen, wishing she could eavesdrop on the discussion but knowing that, for some reason, Jarrett wanted a new confidant right then. He deserved a private conversation.

Jarrett told Rick he did not want to play games this day. He lifted his shirt and showed Rick his surgery scars. He said "My time is almost up. They can't do anything else."

Then he asked Rick to get a piece of paper. He said "I want you to help me make a list."

It was to be a to-do list of things Jarrett wanted to accomplish in the days leading up to his death and things he wanted his parents to do after he was gone.

There were some private messages in the list, things his parents don't want to share. They will always be special because they were love notes for them and his grandmothers, not meant for anyone else to see. But at the top of the list was a simple plea: "Prepare Claire."

Jarrett was concerned about how his sister would go on without him. He wanted to make sure his parents talked to her about what was soon to happen. He feared all of the attention had been on his feelings and that Claire would be the one who needed counseling more. He was not wrong. The Mynears did spend time talking to their daughter about how Jarrett would soon go to a better place where he would no longer be in pain. They told her Jarrett wanted her to be happy for him, and she promised she would try.

Or course, Jarrett's list included "Keep the Joy Cart rolling."

The other bullet point that stood out was "Do something to make the clinic better." Specifically, he asked his mom to try to get new furniture for the clinic and also get some video game systems. He named some people he believed would make a donation. It was obvious he had been thinking about this for some time.

When Jarrett finished dictating the list to Rick, the boy drifted back to sleep. Rick handed the sheet of paper to Jennifer, who told him, "Now you get it, right? This is the way he needed to open up to you. You just needed to wait on his timing."

She put the list in a safe place, but within easy reach.

Three days later, October 3rd, Jarrett was so weak he could not hold his head up. He was unable to eat. Now, the Mynears truly felt helpless and hopeless. Nurse Anne Hoskins came to the house to sit with Jarrett and his parents, trying to keep the boy comfortable and the family composed. Jarrett lay on the couch, drifting in and out of sleep and in and out of conversations. The hours seemed long, yet each minute was precious. Just after dinner time, another favorite nurse, Barb Waldman-Ward came to relieve Anne. The two nurses, who had become dear family friends, were determined one of them would stay with Jarrett until the end.

Nurse Barb, sitting on the floor with her back against the couch in the Mynears' living room, held Jarrett's hand. Doug and Jennifer sat in chairs nearby, trying to make small talk about the weather or local news, anything to keep them all from breaking down in front of their son.

Late in the evening, Jarrett pointed to his parents and asked them to go to the end of the couch. He asked Nurse Barb to hand him the digital camera that was sitting on an end table. It was heavy for him. Barb helped him hold it steady.

"Put your arms around each other," Jarrett said, with a voice that was barely a whisper. His parents managed to smile.

With shaky hands, he snapped a picture.

"There," he smiled. "That's what I needed."

Tears welled up in the eyes of both Jennifer and Doug. Nurse Barb also fought back tears as she took the camera from Jarrett's hands. The one-shot photo shoot was a special moment, as if Jarrett had just imprinted a lasting image in his mind of the two people he loved the most—the mom and dad who had helped him focus on positive things throughout a life of struggle, pain, setbacks, and celebrations. Those words, "That's what I needed," seemed so simple yet profound.

"Now, you all have to get some sleep," Barb told Doug and Jennifer. "You're exhausted. Please go to bed. I'm not going anywhere."

So they did as they were told, leaving the nurse and their son alone in the living room.

"They talked off and on throughout the night," Jennifer said. "I don't know everything they talked about."

But she does know Barb was a calming presence for everyone in the house.

The next morning, after a restless night, Jennifer tiptoed down to the kitchen to fix a cup of coffee. She carried it to the living room, where Jarrett was asleep. Nurse Barb was still there on the floor, awake and holding his hand. Jennifer went to the end table to look at the photo on the camera's memory card. It was a pretty good picture of her and Doug. Somehow, despite having tumors in his brain that pressed on his optic nerves and affected his vision, Jarrett had managed to get the shot centered. Jennifer broke down when she noticed how Jarrett's red, swollen feet framed the bottom corners of the picture, evidence that he couldn't lift the camera quite high enough. She and Doug loved that little photographer and will always cherish his captured moment. It's not a cliché to Jennifer when she says that picture is worth a thousand words.

Anne stopped back by the house that morning and everyone agreed the time had come to take Jarrett to the hospital. When he tried to speak, many of his words made no sense. He had once told his parents he did not want to die at home.

As they were getting things in order, another friend knocked on the door. Marilyn Bryant was the mother of one of Jarrett's school friends. She was just popping in to say hello. She had no idea how dire things were until she walked in and was devastated by her bad timing.

Marilyn realized immediately she had to make this a quick visit and tried to keep Jarrett from sensing how her heart had just broken. Before excusing herself, she asked Jarrett if she could do anything for him.

"A root beer float," the boy whispered.

Marilyn managed the A&W restaurant in Nicholasville, one of Jarrett's favorite hangouts.

"That's easy," Marilyn said. "I'll be right back."

She hurried away and drove straight to the restaurant, which was just five miles away. She unlocked the doors and made a float as quickly as she could. She got back to the house just as the family was pulling out of the driveway.

Jarrett managed to take a few sips of the frothy drink as they drove to the hospital.

When they arrived, the nurses met the family in the hospital parking garage. The caregivers had a gurney waiting, piled with pillows and blankets to cushion Jarrett's frail body as they whisked him to an awaiting room.

Doug and Jennifer stayed by Jarrett's bedside all afternoon and into the evening. Some other family members and close friends came to sit with them. One of them who was staying at the house with Claire brought her to the hospital long enough for her to give her brother a hug and kiss. I stopped by briefly on my dinner break, along with my now-married co-anchor, Jennifer Nime Palumbo. Jarrett may not have been aware of our presence, yet we were drawn to see him one more time and whisper encouragement to him.

From time to time, Jarrett mumbled some words that no one could understand, but his last words were loud and clear. Just as it was turning dark outside, and inside that room, the boy turned his head toward his parents and said, "Thank you. I love you."

Word of Jarrett's death spread quickly. It was difficult for me to report it on the newscast that night, but Jarrett was a public figure and viewers would want to know. We had a lot of file tape, and it was easy to edit together a quick obituary. But this was personal. I had lost a friend. When we broke for commercials, my co-anchor and I both wiped away tears.

Three days later, a line of people snaked out the front door of the funeral home and into the parking lot for the visitation. It was nearly a three-hour wait to reach Jarrett's parents to share condolences. Doug and Jennifer stood next to an easel displaying a large photo of a smiling Jarrett surrounded by toys. That was the only way most people had ever seen him. Officers from the Lexington police department stood on each side of the closed casket, serving as honor guards. The casket contained items dear to Jarrett, including Raggedy Andy, who was listed in Jarrett's obituary as a constant companion, and a rod and reel placed there by his fishing buddy, Uncle Chris. Milt Hettinger, a Louisville firefighter and rescue squad member who conducted scuba diving lessons each year for the children at Indian Summer Camp, asked to pin a medal of valor on Jarrett's shirt. Milt had been awarded the medal for saving a life but told the Mynears Jarrett deserved it, noting the definition of valor is "heroic courage."

Dozens of strangers joined the receiving line, people whom the Mynears didn't know but who wanted to show their respect and tell them how they had been inspired by their son's strength and generosity.

At the funeral on October 8th, the Rev. Linh Nguyen reminded 600 mourners at Mary Queen of the Holy Rosary Church that Jarrett would want them to be happy for him.

"He was a Wonder Boy who taught us to love as a kid loves," the priest said, noting that Jarrett was not impressed by power or prestige and that he did not notice race, religious denomination, or gender. "St. Paul calls us all children of God."

"Jarrett had a passion to take away the pain of other children," Nguyen eulogized. "He wanted us to remember that it's with a simple toy that children sit together and play. There we find Christ; there we find common peace and love."

The priest reminded the listeners how once Jarrett set his mind to a project, he had the tenacity to see it through to the end—how his dogged determination would turn a "no" into a "yes."

"Don't be sad today," he said, grinning at the boy's parents. "Have joy because Jarrett is no longer harassing you. He is harassing God right now!"

In one of the funeral's most moving moments, the priest told the congregation that Jarrett was a great kid because he had great parents. "Doug and Jennifer," he said, "You are what made him what he was."

The congregation rose in unison to give the Mynears an extended standing ovation.

Jennifer's brother, Christopher Wagner, read a poem she had written that was a promise to carry on Jarrett's message. Her other brother, Michael, spoke on the family's behalf, thanking those in attendance for their support over the years.

The sermon ended with a moment Jarrett would have loved. Father Linh lifted up a giant super soaker Jarrett had given him as a gift months earlier. The priest stood behind Jarrett's casket, pumped the water gun's handle and sprayed the crowd. Laughter rang through the church. That was the right way to remember a boy who never wanted anyone to shed tears for him.

The procession of cars that followed the hearse to Lexington Cemetery went on for miles. Drivers noticed signs on business marquees along the way that read "Rest in Peace, Jarrett Mynear." The route went past a section of High Street, which two years earlier city leaders had ceremoniously given the second, honorary name, "Jarrett Mynear Way."

When the procession entered the gates of Lexington Cemetery, four police officers stood at attention: two on horseback, one standing with a dog and one with a bicycle, representing different patrol units. Members of the SWAT (Special Weapons and Tactics) team were also there. The police loved Jarrett and wanted to treat him as a fallen officer. At the gravesite, they fired off a 15-gun salute in the boy's honor.

Applause, laughter, gunfire! Jarrett had wanted every day to be special and even his funeral day was extraordinary.

A Poem for Jarrett
by Jennifer Mynear

Longing arms, aching heart,
The end of a life just at its start.
Gaping hole exists inside;
Make us want to run and hide.
Hide from the heart bewilderment and pain
'Til we're together in Heaven again.
The joys were many, the years were brief,
A flood of memories, pray, temper the grief.
The arms that long to hold you near,
Flesh of our flesh, our child so dear.
Your time is over,
Your mark true and strong.
We will carry your message
Our whole lives long.

46

Marching Orders

The days that followed were sad for the family, of course. Even though the house was full of casseroles and cakes friends had brought over, no one felt much like eating. Emotions ran the gamut from happy memories to deep grief.

By Saturday, Jennifer found herself alone, aimlessly picking up items around the house and putting dishes away. She had trouble keeping her mind on any one task. She straightened up some cards and papers on the desk in her kitchen. When she opened the top drawer, there was the list: Jarrett's final wishes.

It was the spark she needed to get her to focus on the future. The Joy Cart had missed a Tuesday night run for just the second time since it started because of Jarrett's funeral. But the list said "Keep the Joy Cart rolling." She had always intended to do that, but had she made arrangements for the coming Tuesday? She picked up the phone and called some loyal volunteers to make sure they were on the schedule. Jennifer needed a little more time to pass before she would feel like going back into the hospital—just a week or two—but that was no reason for the toy deliveries to be put on hold. The patients would be disappointed. In fact, she reminded herself nurses had seen children cry because they were getting dismissed from the hospital on a Monday, meaning they would miss the Tuesday ritual.

Then, there was that bigger item on Jarrett's list: "Do something to make the clinic better." The words hit his mom like a marching order. She could almost hear his voice, saying "Well, what are you waiting for?"

She decided she would get right on it Monday morning. It would be just the thing she needed to lift her spirits.

Just before Jarrett's death, Dr. Moscow was also thinking about ways to make the clinic better, and some fundraising had begun. He, Jennifer, and Jarrett had often talked about how the clinic needed a makeover. Moscow's son played in a band with the son of the woman who oversaw development at UK's Markey Cancer Center. When he got to know Susannah Denomme through that musical link, Moscow told her the clinic really needed help, and he told her about Jarrett. She knew about The Joy Cart through news accounts, but had no personal connection to it.

"He said, 'I want you to meet Jennifer,'" Susannah recalled. "He called her a 'force of nature.'" But the timing wasn't right. Jarrett was just too ill.

So, Susannah was one of those strangers in the receiving line at the funeral home the night before Jarrett was buried. She stood in line with Dr. Moscow for nearly three hours, nervously approaching a family in mourning. "I didn't feel equal to the occasion," she said. "But Dr. Moscow wanted me to see what an impact this little boy had had."

She saw the photos and read newspaper clippings on display as she waited, and it did give her a better understanding of Jarrett's influence—a realization that his life had been about more than giving away toys.

Jennifer does not remember meeting Susannah at the funeral home. The whole experience of greeting guests alongside her son's casket is a blurry memory. But she does remember liking her immediately when Dr. Moscow brought her to the house a week later. The two, who were about the same age and who had attended UK at the same time, just clicked.

Like her son, Jennifer did not take things slowly. Before that first meeting ended, plans were made to establish The Jarrett Mynear Fund with the sole purpose of renovating the pediatric cancer clinic as soon as possible.

"When Jarrett made his list, he didn't have a new clinic in mind," Jennifer said. "He just thought we should get some nice chairs and some video game systems. But we all wanted to do more and thought the time was right."

Jennifer was also cautious. Although the fund bore Jarrett's name, she didn't want him to become a billboard just for the purpose of fundraising. "She was very protective of how we used his name and image in promoting the fund," Susannah said. "She wanted to make sure this was being done in honor of all the clinic's patients, past and present."

In the month after the funeral, $70,000 came in from donors who gave money for the clinic in lieu of flowers. That was a grand start. Jennifer called on Dream Factory contacts, business owners, and bankers she had met over the years, asking all of them to think of ways to boost the fund. Over the next several months, there were so many events planned, Jennifer and Susannah had a difficult time getting them all on the calendar.

There were silent auctions, golf scrambles, bake sales, and a motorcycle rally. The Lexington Rotary Club raised money with a Valentine's Day dance. A hair salon had a brunch and donated all the proceeds from one day's styling appointments to the fund. Ron Turner, the man who had purchased the go-cart for Jarrett years before, sponsored a fundraising luncheon.

In all, $750,000 was raised for the renovation, with $400,000 coming directly from The Jarrett Mynear Fund. A check for $150,000 came from The Makenna Foundation, another nonprofit organization in Lexington formed in memory of a child. McKenna David, a former patient at the UK clinic, was just twenty months old when she died in 1998 of a rare lung disorder. Since Jarrett's death, the two funds have often worked together.

On April 12, 2005, the new University of Kentucky Pediatric Hematology-Oncology Clinic opened in the same location as the old clinic, but at 3,000 square feet, it was twice as big as its predecessor. Dr. Moscow called it the nicest pediatric facility he had ever seen. It featured the state's first outpatient pediatric sedation center, private family rooms for infusions, and its own laboratory and pharmacy. The waiting area had two new computers families could use to access information about illnesses and treatments.

The former facility had just eight seats for children undergoing blood transfusions or chemotherapy. Often caretakers and parents had to sit on the floor to be near their young patients. The new center had fifteen seats. And, of course, there were new gaming systems the patients could use in the treatment room to make their time there more bearable. And a big screen TV. It was Jarrett's wish fulfilled and so much more.

47

Ripples

Jarrett's Joy Cart was the big splash that started the Mynears on a path of giving and patient advocacy. It's what drew TV cameras to the hospital and prompted invitations for Jarrett to appear on national talk shows. It's what made him a celebrity.

But when you jump in a pool, the splash makes ripples that touch other people. Jarrett's jump was like doing a cannonball. It caused a lot of other people to get drenched in the desire to do good.

It was a Sunday school handout that lit a fire under nine-year-old Ethan Hampton of Festus, Missouri. One Sunday in the summer of 2002, he came out of his class at First United Methodist Church, eager to show his mother an article in the weekly reader his teacher had passed out. The lesson was about helping others, with Jarrett's Joy Cart featured as an example.

"Mom, we need to help this boy," Ethan said, even before they had left the sanctuary that morning.

Debbie and Wade Hampton were delighted that their son was showing a desire to be generous, so that afternoon Debbie did some research. She googled "Jarrett's Joy Cart" and found a wealth of information on the Internet.

Over the next few weeks, she called come area hospitals to see if they would allow her son to come in and distribute toys.

"The local hospitals turned us down," Debbie said. "Volunteers had to be at least sixteen years old. That was an unbendable rule at the first three hospitals I contacted."

But Ethan told her to keep trying. Debbie set her sights a little farther from home and called Cardinal Glennon Children's Hospital, which was forty-five minutes away in St. Louis.

"The public relations manager there loved the idea of kids helping kids," Debbie said. "She said, 'If Ethan brings us toys, we'll make sure he gets to deliver them to patients.'"

So Debbie wrote a letter outlining what Ethan wanted to do, and he signed it. They sent fifty copies of it to friends, relatives, and members of their church. And just like with Jarrett's cart, donations poured in right way.

In October, Ethan made his first room-to-room visits at the hospital. Unlike Jarrett, Ethan was not sick and had never been in a hospital for a serious reason.

"He just had a lot of compassion," his mother said. And he believed he was helping Jarrett expand his dream, even though the Hamptons and Mynears had never met or even talked on the phone.

"He called it 'Jarrett's Joy Cart' at first," Debbie said. "But that was confusing. The patients thought Ethan was Jarrett, and they thought he was sick. We changed the sign on the cart to say 'Joy Cart by Ethan' but always told patients we got the idea from a boy in Kentucky."

When Jennifer learned of the Missouri cart, she was delighted and considered it even more special because the Hamptons had done it on their own. "Our hands weren't in it," Jennifer said, "but Jarrett's spirit definitely was.

Like Jarrett, Ethan was interviewed on television and featured in newspaper articles. That fueled the effort. Toys "R" Us sent him a $1,000 gift card, and his church served as a collection point for money and toys. The Missouri Highway Patrol had a toy drive that resulted in truckloads of donations.

Debbie's parents stored the toys in their unfinished basement and had to build shelves along the walls so they could get some order to the operation.

Shortly after Ethan's first run, Jarrett died. Ethan took the news hard, but it also made him more resolved to make as many deliveries to the hospital as he could.

Ethan's Joy Cart ran twice a month for nearly three years. It began to wind down when he was in the fifth grade. "I had to pull him out of school each time we needed to be in St. Louis for a delivery. The school was great about it, but as Ethan got more involved in other activities, both during and after school, it became more difficult for us to schedule deliveries on a regular basis."

Debbie points to those joy cart years as the most important ones of Ethan's life. The project showed him that giving is infectious. He was amazed by how many people wanted to help him. And it prompted his sister Renae to embrace Operation Christmas Child, the annual international relief project coordinated by Samaritan's Purse. The Hamptons say they couldn't count how many shoeboxes Renae has filled with small toys, hygiene items and school supplies to be sent to impoverished children around the world. But they know Ethan's happiness in giving was a major influence on his sister.

In the spring of 2002, Jessica Abo, through Northwestern University's Medill School of Journalism, was assigned to an internship in our newsroom in Lexington. I could tell right away she had a heart for philanthropy. She told me how even as a high school student she had led efforts to raise money for good causes. And she had a desire to report good news and stories about the human spirit. I was eager for her to learn about Jarrett's Joy Cart.

Jessica went back to Chicago that summer and read an earlier version of this book, "just to be nice" to me, she said. "But I was blown away by what I read," she said. "I had never been so touched by a story in my life."

She e-mailed Jennifer and told her she wanted to try to start a Joy Cart in Illinois. Even though it was out of the blue and she had no idea who Jessica was, Jennifer could sense this 19-year-old girl was serious and determined. But Jarrett had taken a turn for the worse, and the Mynears had a lot on their plate. They didn't give Jessica's proposal too much thought at the time.

Jarrett died a few weeks after that initial contact. Jessica felt compelled to get in her car and make the eight-hour drive to Lexington. She met the Mynears face-to-face for the first time at the funeral home.

"I was devastated that I never had a chance to talk to Jarrett, to let him know that I was working on his dream of getting more joy carts started."

The outpouring of love she saw for Jarrett that weekend gave her the final push she needed. The next weekend, Jessica ran the Chicago Marathon, wearing a yellow ribbon in Jarrett's memory.

Then she was off and running with the project, enlisting the help of Northwestern Hillel, the foundation for Jewish student life on campus.

"We pounded the pavement to find partners," she said, marveling at how she randomly made contact with a man who owned a toy distribution warehouse. "He wanted to stay anonymous but told me to come in and pick out anything we needed."

That man donated hundreds of toys over the months that followed.

Through perseverance, Jessica got permission to run Jarrett's NU Joy Cart through the halls of Evanston Northwestern Hospital on a weekly basis, starting in April 2003. There was a lot of red tape to get past to make it happen, but, like Jarrett, this young dynamo wouldn't take "no" for an answer.

Months later, Jessica also inspired students at an elementary school in Marlboro, New Jersey, to form their own version of a joy cart. The Mynears have given their blessing to each one of Jessica's efforts, impressed by her energy and ability to make things happen.

Now, as an author and motivational speaker, Jessica often tells young people about Jarrett's Joy Cart. During a 2013 speech to one thousand teenagers in New Orleans, she offered to write college recommendation letters for anyone who created a project around the idea of spreading joy. Many students ran with the challenge, doing such things as working to make a playground more accessible to children with disabilities and bringing live music performances to the residents of a nursing home.

"I'm always hoping Jarrett is looking down on me," Jessica said. "I hope he sees a girl he never met who wants to carry his flag."

Leah Nash was diagnosed with leukemia in 2008 when she was four years old and spent many long weeks at the University of Kentucky Children's Hospital. Her treatment lasted two years, so she was in and out of the hospital a lot and had several Tuesday visits from Jarrett's Joy Cart. Her parents, Sarah and Robert Nash, said it always brightened her day.

"On days she was admitted, it became the kind of thing where she'd immediately say, 'Is this Tuesday?'" her mom laughed.

Leah always picked arts and crafts items from the cart.

Five months after her treatments ended, she relapsed. The next move for her was a trip to Cincinnati Children's Hospital for a bone marrow transplant. While recovering, Leah began to ask her mom about The Joy Cart, recalling how it had made her so happy. That's when Sarah looked into the cart's backstory and told her daughter about Jarrett.

Leah, then seven years old, decided she wanted to help. She told her mom she was going to raise $1,000 and give it to Jarrett's Joy Cart. Her mother said that was a lofty goal but gave the spunky girl permission to try.

Leah had no qualms about going door to door in her neighborhood to ask for donations. She got a couple hundred dollars that way.

"Now what?" she wondered. Her family was about to have a yard sale, so she decided to set up a table of her own items, with her income going to the cart. And she sold lemonade and cookies, too.

That went better than expected and got her closer to the goal because many people purposely overpaid for their purchases when they found out why Leah was raising money. Leah set up a lemonade stand in front of their home many more weekends that summer and fall and the next summer, too. When she had $1,000, her mother called Jennifer to tell her what Leah had done.

"I was speechless," Jennifer said. "I didn't know she was doing that and couldn't believe it when I heard how determined she was to help."

It was impossible for Jennifer to remember all of the thousands of young patients she had met on Joy Cart runs over the years, but certain ones stood out. Leah was one of them. Even when Leah was very sick, she had always greeted the cart volunteers with a big smile and words of gratitude.

Over the phone, Sarah asked Jennifer if Leah could meet her and deliver the money personally.

"I had a better idea," Jennifer said. "I asked Leah if she would like to go with me on a shopping spree to pick out toys for the cart."

Leah jumped at the chance and showed up in the parking lot of Lexington's Toys "R" Us with cash in hand. She untied a ribbon from around a pink plastic container and opened it to show Jennifer a huge stack of mostly one dollar bills.

"Let's go!" she giggled with excitement.

Over the next two hours, they filled up four shopping carts.

Jennifer said it was wonderful having Leah along. She took great care in deciding what toys would be good for the cart. She really helped Jennifer determine what the new "cool" toys kids wanted were.

"It was fun for me," Leah said. "I knew some kids who were still in the hospital, and I thought about how much they would enjoy getting certain things I picked out. I liked being able to help them in that way."

Leah enjoyed helping the cart so much she decided she was going to do it again with a goal twice as large. She spent another two summers setting up more yard sales and lemonade stands. By then, her family was funneling all yard sale profits into Leah's fund. And she also began selling her hand-drawn artwork through an online store she had set up on Etsy. Visitors to the *ArtistsPlaceShop* on that site can still find pictures of flowers and cartoon characters selling for $10 or $15, with proceeds clearly earmarked for Jarrett's Joy Cart.

Leah reached that $2,000 goal and has had more since then, each one a little greater than the last. She said she doesn't see herself ever stopping. With Toys "R" Us out of business, her shopping sprees may now spread out over several stores. She looks forward to her 18th birthday when she will be allowed on the patient floors at the Kentucky Children's Hospital to push The Joy Cart herself.

In 2009, when Steven and Allison Scrivner began planning a third birthday party for their daughter Paige, they decided they did not want her friends to bring gifts. Paige had a house full of toys and would get plenty more from her parents and grandparents when the special day arrived.

"In fact," Paige's dad said, "we were looking for ways to put some of the toys she already had to good use." Like all kids, Paige had her favorite toys and there were others she never played with.

The Scrivners lived near the Mynears and knew about Jarrett's Joy Cart. They decided they would ask the people coming to the party to bring a toy after all, but for the cart rather than for their daughter.

"We are fortunate people," Steven said. "We wanted Paige to realize that not everyone has as many things as she does and that it feels good to help them."

That began a tradition of collecting donations for The Joy Cart each year when Paige's birthday rolled around.

"When she was five and six years old, she didn't necessarily buy into it completely," her dad said. "Sometimes someone would bring a gift as a donation that was something Paige was reluctant to give away. We had to explain to her that the toys were going to really sick children who were stuck in the hospital."

They helped her paint a picture in her mind of how a child might react when he or she saw a certain toy on a cart rolled into their hospital room.

"We wanted to instill in her, and later, her younger brother Easton, the idea of philanthropy and helping others."

By Paige's seventh birthday, she was all on board. By then she saw it as a challenge to see how many toys she could collect and give away. A couple days after that year's party, the Scrivners filled up the back of their family van and drove to the Mynears house to deliver the toys.

"Doug and Jennifer treated her as if she had done the greatest thing in the world," Steven said. "They told her she had a big heart."

They hugged Paige and took pictures of her with the toys to put on The Joy Cart's Facebook page. Jennifer told her she was setting a good example and that one day she would be old enough to push the cart in the hospital and see firsthand what a difference she was making.

As Paige has grown older, her birthday parties have grown larger, moving away from the family home to rented facilities such as a roller skating rink. Her friends all know a big part of the party is to build a mountain of toys for The Joy Cart, and they seem to take pride in their gift giving, putting a lot of thought into what would make a child happy in the hospital.

The parties spilled into another annual event for the Scrivners, who are big University of Kentucky football fans. They love the game day ritual of tailgating for hours before kickoff in the parking lot outside the stadium.

In 2006, when Paige was just a few weeks old, the family was tailgating in a grassy area near the stadium when a sudden storm came up. The rain clouds parked over the stadium and dumped a huge amount of rain in a small area. In a matter of minutes, lower lying areas around the stadium became a fast-flowing river. The flash flood covered cars with water and swept tents and tables into storm sewers. Drenched fans rushed for higher ground.

It was a freak act of nature, but the abrupt storm laid the groundwork for another flood of donations—one that would spring up a few years later.

The flooding forced the university to close off parking in the sunken areas outside the stadium, so the Scrivners relocated their tailgate parties to another lot. They found a spot next to Ralph Coldiron, the past president of The Dream Factory, who had helped arrange Jarrett's shopping spree at Best Buy eleven years earlier. The Scrivners routinely drew 40 to 50 people to their parking lot party each home game; so did Ralph. So the merged tailgate setups often attracted more than a hundred people.

Ralph and Steven picked a game late in the season and announced they would be having a chili cook-off. That drew the biggest crowd they had ever had visit their joint pregame celebration.

The next season, people kept asking the two of them if they were going to do a chili cook-off again.

"I told Ralph if we did it, we should try to help out a good cause too," Steven said. Ralph agreed, and the pair didn't have to think long about what that cause would be.

"We invited friends to come and told them they could eat as much as they wanted for free, as long as they brought a toy for Jarrett's Joy Cart," Steven said.

It was a success. Now, each fall, the tailgate chili cook-off brings in about 150 toys. Paige Scrivner is right there to greet the generous football fans who come to the party, eager to relieve them of their packages and hand them a bowl.

When Jennifer speaks to church or civic groups about The Joy Cart, she emphasizes that the toys are a way to make an emotional connection. There is proof the toys are not cast aside and forgotten. Many families have told her how a visit from The Joy Cart has become a lifelong fond memory.

One Tuesday evening shortly after Jarrett's death, Jennifer was steering the "baby cart" past the intensive care unit at the University of Kentucky Children's Hospital. It's the cart loaded down with items for patients three years old and younger. The top shelf was completely covered by one item—a huge yellow stuffed duck someone had donated.

"It was the fluffiest thing you've ever seen, "Jennifer said. "All of the volunteers wanted to rub it. But it was so big you couldn't put your arms around it."

It caught the eye of a mother who spied it through the glass window of the ICU. She rushed out to stop the cart.

"I know my son is a teenager," she told Jennifer, "but is there any way I could have that duck?"

Jennifer laughed and asked her if she was sure her son would want it. She saw the woman's boy in a bed through the window. He was a big, husky guy.

"The cart for teenagers will be coming by next, "Jennifer told the woman. "You might want to see what we have on it this week."

The mother insisted her son T. J. would love to have the duck. She said he had a much smaller version of the same duck when he was a toddler and that he had loved it, but he had lost it years ago and they had never been able to replace it. The boy was in a coma, and the mother said she would love for him to see the duck when he came out of it.

Of course, Jennifer said she could have it. The mother placed the duck at the foot of her son's bed.

The next Tuesday when The Joy Cart rolled around again, that same mom met Jennifer in a hallway and hugged her.

"My son came out of the coma the day after your last visit," the mother said. "He opened his eyes and the first thing he said was, 'My duck grew!'"

Jennifer looked in the window of the ICU, and the boy was there. He waved and smiled at her, with the stuffed animal by his side.

Eighteen months later, Jennifer was called to be a substitute teacher in a high school classroom. To break the ice, she wanted to tell the students a little about herself and then go around the room and have the students tell an interesting fact from their own lives.

Jennifer told the students she had once been a full-time teacher, but now she spent most of her time running a project called "Jarrett's Joy Cart."

A large boy in the back of the room stopped her. "I know you," he said, "You're the duck lady!"

Jennifer didn't realize what he was talking about at first. So, the boy continued.

"I was in the hospital, and you gave me a big fluffy duck."

Some of the other teens in the room started laughing. But the boy, who looked big enough to win any fight, shot them a look that made them go silent.

"It was important to me, and I still have it," he said.

Then Jennifer remembered the encounter and continued telling the class about The Joy Cart, now with the perfect example of how little things can make a big difference to some people.

Four years later, Jennifer was going down a hall in another part of the hospital when a familiar-looking woman approached her.

"Please may I give you a hug?" the woman asked. "I can't believe I get to see you again. You may not remember me, but you gave my son a big duck when he was in intensive care."

Jennifer assured her that she did remember and told her how special it was to her that her son thanked her when he was a student in one of her classes.

"Well, I want you to know something else," the mother said. "T. J. will be a daddy in a few weeks. That duck is sitting in the nursery waiting on that baby boy!"

After attending Jarrett's funeral in 2002, Doug's former college roommate, Albert Cooper, just could not get it out of his mind. He was so impressed by the way the community had supported Jarrett's Joy Cart and what an impact it was still making on so many people.

So, unbeknownst to the Mynears, Al and his wife Lisa began talking to administrators at Florida Hospital in Orlando near where they lived about starting a Joy Cart there.

"We just wanted to honor Jarrett's dream of having Joy Carts all across the country," Al said. As he remembers it, it was an easy sell to get the hospital to agree to it.

He made sure they did everything correctly, setting up the cart as a nonprofit organization and providing the proper documentation to the hospital.

On April 8, 2003, just a week before what would have been Jarrett's 13th birthday, the hospital paid to fly the Mynears to Orlando for a ribbon-cutting ceremony for the fourth official Jarrett's Joy Cart.

That cart ran once a month, and the Coopers estimate they gave out more than 5,000 toys before the project ended in 2012. Al says the recession caused the cart to come to an end.

"We were a mom-and-pop charity, and it became tough to compete with other charities for donations and volunteers," he said. "We just didn't want to keep tapping our friends for donations."

Al, an architect, also had a job change and had to spend nearly a year back in Kentucky, which made it difficult to keep managing the charity from afar.

But the Coopers see those nine years as a highlight of their lives. They believe it molded their daughters, Lauren and Amy, into more compassionate people with a lasting desire to help others.

Jennifer's mantra that the cart is about making connections really hit home with Lisa one day when she came across a toddler in the hall of the hospital.

"I asked her grandmother, who was with her, if the little girl would like to pick a toy off the cart," Lisa said. "But the grandmother said the girl couldn't do it because she was blind."

Lisa immediately thought of a toy that was on another cart in a different part of the hospital and told the grandmother to wait for her to come back.

"It was a caterpillar with tactile segments," Lisa said. "One segment was crunchy, another was velvety to the touch—that sort of thing.

"I've never forgotten the look on that little girl's face after I gave her that caterpillar. She lit up as she worked her hands over each segment."

To Lisa, it was like magic to pair a child with the perfect toy. "Magic" is a word that has often been used to describe Jarrett's Joy Cart.

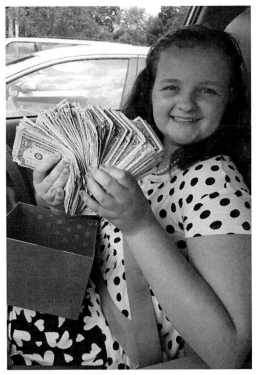

Leah Nash prepares to go on a shopping spree for Jarrett's Joy Cart

48

No Time to Rest

After the new University of Kentucky Pediatric Hematology-Oncology Clinic opened in 2005, it would have been a good time for the Mynears to get some rest. They had been involved in fundraising projects almost nonstop for the past six years. But Jennifer wasn't finished—not by a long shot. Other plans were already in motion.

The new clinic was a dream come true, but it would need sustaining funds and it could still use more equipment and more staff. The clinic's workload had increased 35 percent from a decade earlier. At any given time, about 100 children were at some stage of chemotherapy treatment.

Susannah Denomme had moved into a new position at the university. As the Associate Vice President for Philanthropy, she was now charged with finding donors for a multitude of programs and projects on campus. However, she wasn't about to let the clinic be pushed down the priority list.

She and Jennifer had talked about what should happen next, even before the clinic renovation was completed. They both agreed they would like to get students involved. Frankly, they needed their energy and enthusiasm. Enrollment topped 25,000 that year. Surely those students were an underutilized resource.

But what would get students excited? Susannah and Jennifer brainstormed, but none of their ideas seemed big enough. How many students would be committed to a carnival, scavenger hunts or a Valentine's Day dance? Susannah asked her daughter Carolyn, who was a student at Penn State University, if she had any ideas. She did not have to think long at all. She told her mom to go online and check out "THON." It's the largest student-run philanthropy in the world, an annual year-long effort to raise money for pediatric cancer care that wraps up each February with a 46-hour-long dance marathon. Carolyn told her mother THON had been a unifying event on campus for more than 30 years and was bringing in more than ten million dollars annually!

Jennifer and Susannah both went home and did some research. They perused dozens of articles and photographs on their home computers. Each click of the keyboard made them more excited about the possibilities. When they met again a few days later at Starbucks, they were both energized to present the idea to student leaders on campus.

"This could be huge," Jennifer told Susannah. "I just wonder if we can pull it off."

A barista called Susannah's name at the counter. When she picked up her hot coffee, a chill ran through her body. The cardboard band around the cup seemed to be sending a message. She turned the cup so Jennifer could read it: "Always Remember the Dance."

In late 2004, Jennifer and Susannah met with leaders of student government, the Panhellenic Council, the student activities board, and student volunteer organization. Each young person they met with liked the idea of a campus-wide event focused on philanthropy and worked to get the word out about an open meeting in the student center. More than 100 students came to the informational session.

Mark Denomme, Susannah's husband, worked in the Information Technology department at UK. He showed the attendees a video presentation he had put together featuring highlights from THON. Jennifer talked about how Jarrett's Joy Cart had brought her to this point.

"I was surprised how many students had heard of Jarrett," she said. "It was now two years past his death, and he had long been out of the news. But I found out some of the students in that room had once been patients at the children's hospital and had received toys from the cart."

A show of hands indicated the students wanted to pursue the dance event.

Susannah told them there would be another meeting soon and at that time she wanted students to take control of the project. "Be prepared to elect officers, form committees and run with it," she said. "This is yours to do with it what you will. We'll help, but you don't have to worry about any of us micromanaging your decisions."

As Susannah and Jennifer left the room and headed down a hallway, they heard footsteps coming up quickly behind them.

"I'm glad I caught you," a voice said. "I just know I'm supposed to help with this."

It was Emily Pfeiffer, a junior finance major from Columbus, Ohio. She had just lived through some stressful months, and a big project seemed to her to be just the thing she needed to regain her focus.

Emily had been diagnosed with thyroid cancer the summer before, but most of her friends didn't know about it. And her father was unexpectedly diagnosed with stage four liver cancer at the same time.

"Cancer is such a scary word," she said. "I felt fortunate that my treatment was over and had gone so well, but my father was growing weaker each day. My desire to help was influenced by that."

Two weeks later, Emily interviewed to be the overall chair of the event and got the job.

Another student who wanted the job was Amberlee Kempf, a sophomore design major from Hebron, Connecticut. She heard about the project through the Office of Student Involvement.

"It just struck a chord with me," she said. "In high school, I lost a friend to pediatric cancer, and this call to arms made me want to step up."

She said that, until she met Emily, she was disappointed she had not been selected as the overall chair.

"She was perfect for the job, and we became like sisters."

Amberlee was chosen to be the head of dancer programming, a position she quickly embraced. That meant she would choreograph a line dance for all participants to learn and come up with a theme for each hour of the marathon. She was comfortable with that because she had been a cheerleader in middle school and high school.

Participation from sororities and fraternities was key to getting the event off the ground, but Amberlee was not part of that circle. Over the months, however, she says she became "the most Greek non-Greek you'd ever meet." She spent countless hours in the basement of the Chi Omega house working on dance moves with Emily. They would talk and plan until one or both of them fell asleep.

Amberlee is also the one who came up with a name for the event. For weeks, the working name was "Cat-thon" (because the students were all Kentucky Wildcats), but no one really loved the name. Then Amberlee had a better idea.

At that time, the university's head basketball coach, Tubby Smith, was promoting a slogan. He handed out plastic wristbands on campus imprinted with the words "LIVE BLUE." It was a take on professional cyclist Lance Armstrong's LIVESTRONG movement, which had raised tens of millions of dollars for cancer research through the sale of wristbands.

"The mentality on campus was that being blue was a way of conducting yourself," Amberlee said. "It meant you represented your university with pride and dignity."

She presented the name "DanceBlue" to the committee members, who reacted with smiles and relief. Now they had a name they believed would look good on signs, t-shirts, and promotional materials. It had a nice ring to it and meaning, too.

In February 2005, the university paid for plane tickets for Jennifer, Susannah and Emily to fly to Pennsylvania to witness THON. They were accompanied by an advisor from the Office of Student Leadership.

The four of them could not believe how much energy was in that gymnasium on the Penn State campus. Hundreds of students stood shoulder to shoulder on the floor, dancing to videos projected on a huge screen. Each hour, groups would come onto the stage to present giant facsimiles of checks written out in large amounts. They represented monies that had been collected throughout the year at 5-K runs, carnivals, mini-dance marathons, and restaurant promotions. And most impressive of all was the way the students interacted with young cancer patients who were allowed on stage or on the dance floor. No child was ever seen standing alone or lost in the crowd.

Jennifer wondered if the PSU leaders would be receptive to visitors from another university who wanted to copy their idea. That was an unfounded worry.

"The access they gave us was incredible," she said. "They took us behind the scenes, gave us their template, and introduced us to student committee chairs who told us how they divided responsibilities. They realized we were all fighting for the same cause and saw it as a compliment that we would want to spin off of what they did."

The team from Kentucky decided it would not try to reinvent the wheel. The group would tweak what Penn State did and make it work at UK. It decided to stick with a twenty-four-hour event, even though THON goes on for two days. One of Jennifer's biggest concerns was that students would get bored and leave before it was over.

"We really got down to business after that," Emily said. "We decided the first DanceBlue would be in February 2006, which was exactly a year away. But the fundraising and promotion had to start without delay."

Another concern was cost. To jumpstart the project, Jarrett's Joy Cart refrained from making an annual grant request to Children's Charity Fund of the Bluegrass. Jennifer instructed DanceBlue organizers to apply instead. The fund agreed to redirect $10,000 that would have gone to the cart to the marathon, helping it get off the ground.

The bond among the coordinators grew thicker as the planning picked up pace. Susannah's brother died that summer. Amberlee lost her grandmother. Emily's father died in November.

"Having those nights together working on DanceBlue was comforting to all of us," Amberlee said.

"People grieve differently," Emily said. "It was such a hard time for me. DanceBlue was the most positive outlet for my grief. I needed to pour my heart into something positive. DanceBlue helped me as much as it has helped any patient."

In the weeks leading up to the event, the thirty-person committee assigned more specific duties to its subcommittees. There was a group to head up media relations, one to foster relationships with the clinic families, and one to recruit teams of dancers. A technology team was formed to work on a website and social media accounts. And perhaps most importantly, the leaders visited the clinic on a regular basis to see where the money would go. They got to know doctors, nurses, and patients there on a first name basis and really see how deep the needs were.

Emily, Amberlee, and some of the other committee members also made some Tuesday night runs with The Joy Cart. They got to be like members of the Mynear family.

"Jarrett had been so phenomenal," Amberlee said. "And Jennifer believed we could also be phenomenal. She realized if DanceBlue was going to be successful, it had to be student-driven."

Like The Joy Cart, it had to be a labor of love.

About one hundred and seventy students took part in DanceBlue that first year. They didn't really know what they had signed up for. The marathon didn't actually require nonstop dancing, but the rules called for "no sitting/no sleeping." Each hour began with a choreographed line dance that lasted fifteen minutes. It was a student-produced mashup of popular music videos, with movie clips and clinic video mixed in. When the line dance montage was projected on a big screen, students rushed in flash mob fashion to the floor at UK's Memorial Coliseum, spectators rose in the stands, and the energy in the room kicked up several notches. By the end of DanceBlue, participants knew the dance very well. They had done it twenty-four times.

Part of Amberlee's job was to program each hour, making sure there was excitement even in the wee hours of the morning. There was a country music hour, a techno hour, and a Disney hour. Early in the evening, Emily felt a sudden letdown. "I wish we had thought to get glow sticks for the rave hour," she said with regret. "That would've livened things up at 3 A.M."

This is an example of how Doug Mynear contributes in big, unsung ways.

He tracked down Terry Hagan, the Dream Factory board member, and the two of them slipped away from the action to spend a couple hours going to every Walmart and dollar store they could find open to clear their shelves of glow sticks.

When the students weren't dancing, they were often on their feet doing service projects. An assembly line was set up to make peanut butter sandwiches to be distributed to homeless shelters. Other students wrote cards and letters of encouragement for young cancer patients and their families or filled treat bags that would be given to children when they went to the clinic for treatment.

On Sunday morning, there was a memorial hour, when the big screen displayed faces of children who had lost their battles with cancer. It was somber, but also a necessary time for families to come on stage and say thanks to the dancers and to really drive home to the students the importance of their efforts. The boisterous hall was hushed, and many tears flowed as the participants reflected on the purpose behind this big party. Jarrett's story was retold, and Jennifer couldn't help but imagine her son as one of those college students right out there in the thick of the action. It was the kind of thing he would have loved.

The tension broke as the memorial hour morphed into a celebration of life. Dancers were asked to crowd around the stage for a talent show. DanceBlue committee members ushered current clinic patients into the arena. Some of them had shaved heads or missing limbs, but this was now a time to focus on what the kids could do rather than on what they could not— a timeout to take their minds off chemotherapy, blood counts and upcoming surgeries.

Some of the teens and preteens had real talent, as they sang a pop song or showed off dance moves. Those who could not sing or dance were invited up to take part in Nerf gun battles or to hit plastic golf balls into the crowd. Some just paraded across the stage in costumes. It did not matter what they did. Each child was backed up by college students who joined them on stage, acting as their groupies and encouraging them to perform. The dancers treated each child as if he or she were a rock star.

They cheered loudly, chanting as each act ended: "We dance for you. We dance for you. We dance, we dance all night long!"

As the last child came off the stage, UK's fight song blared over the speakers. A volunteer handed each child a trophy and gave out high fives and hugs.

Jennifer and Susannah stood back and watched in amazement. They thought anyone who worried about the current generation would feel a lot better if they could see what was going on in this coliseum.

"It was the most incredible thing I have ever witnessed," Susannah said. "Those students were all about making the world a better place. They saw it as an honor to be on that floor."

The final hour arrived, with very tired college kids finding new strength. They rallied one more time for the line dance, making the last one the best one. The stands were filled again, as spectators who had wandered in and out over the last twenty-four hours returned to be there for the finale. People stood in their seats and danced along.

Emily said the committee had hoped to make $20,000 the first year. She purposely did not keep up with how much money was coming in throughout the marathon. She wanted to be surprised. Committee members lined up in a hallway and were handed large placards with a number on it. They took the stage, and only then did a finance committee member tell them in what order they should stand. They stood, holding the placards upside down at their knees. Anticipation was high on the floor and in the stands as organizers did everything they could to draw out the suspense.

The music got louder, with a drum roll underneath, as the students began to lift their numbers high above their heads, starting on the penny end of the line. The numbers rolled in a wave from right to left as the cheering got louder, revealing the total down to the penny: **$123,323.19.**

It was more than six times what they had hoped for! The crowd burst out chanting "F-T-K . . . F-T-K . . . F-T-K," which means "For The Kids." It is a mantra that is used at similar marathons around the country—a simple phrase that says it all.

The tired but happy dancers left, eager to get some sleep. There would be classes the next morning. But there was still work to be done. The student leaders of the event stayed behind along with Doug and Jennifer Mynear, Mark and Susannah Denomme, and some other dedicated adults. They had to pull tarps up from the floor, haul out leftover food, and put away tables, props, and decorations.

Emily and Amberlee felt great about what had just happened as they rehashed the event while gathering up trash.

"But," Amberlee said. "We can do better. Wait 'til next year!"

DanceBlue has grown into the biggest event on UK's campus. More alumni come back that weekend than return for Homecoming.

In 2013, the total raised topped one million dollars for the first time, and that number has grown every year since. One thousand dancers take to the dance floor each year, a number that would be larger if it did not have to be capped by the fire marshal. Elementary, middle, and high schools across the state hold their own mini-DanceBlue marathons to add to the total.

"DanceBlue came along at just the right time," Amberlee said years later. "That generation wanted to be a part of a tribe. They were Instagram ready, wanting to be part of experiential moments."

She became the overall chair of the event for its second year. She is now married and lives and works as a retail designer in New York City. Emily is raising a family in northern Ohio, where she works as an asset manager. But each February, their hearts, their minds, and often their bodies are back in Lexington.

"Each year when it comes around, I get completely recharged," Amberlee said. "It's a fantastic reminder that there are amazing things going on."

In May 2012, DanceBlue made a commitment to provide one million dollars over four years to build an entirely new outpatient clinic for children with cancer, relocated across the street to be part of the children's hospital. It opened in January 2017 with a new, longer name—one that gives credit where credit is due. It is called the DanceBlue Kentucky Children's Hospital Hematology/Oncology Clinic. At 6,000 square feet, it is a happier-looking place with beach-themed décor. You would never know it is a place where life and death battles take place.

A sailboat full of toys and an illuminated lighthouse are the centerpieces of the play area. A three-hundred-gallon aquarium filled with colorful fish covers one wall. Three computer stations provided by Jarrett's Joy Cart line another wall. That area is dubbed "The Jarrett Mynear Waiting Room."

DanceBlue volunteers visit often to play with patients and their siblings and leave encouraging messages in a wall compartment resembling a "message in a bottle." Jennifer said it is "heart-warming" to know her son and DanceBlue will be forever linked.

"The biggest fear for a parent who has lost a child is that the child will be forgotten," she said. "These students will never know how much of an impact they have had on us and countless others."

DanceBlue money now funds positions the clinic once could not afford.

"When I needed a support group, I was told 'that would be nice, but we don't have the funds for it,'" Jennifer said. "One of the first things they did at this new clinic was to hire a social worker."

Susannah Denomme can recite a long list of things that are possible because of DanceBlue, everything from small "beads of courage" which are given to children as they reach milestones in their treatment to the huge contributions to research, such as studying the effects of chemotherapy on memory and learning.

The annual event has truly transformed pediatric cancer care in Kentucky.

Susannah has misplaced that coffee cup band from 2004, but its simple message still sears in her mind: "Always Remember the Dance."

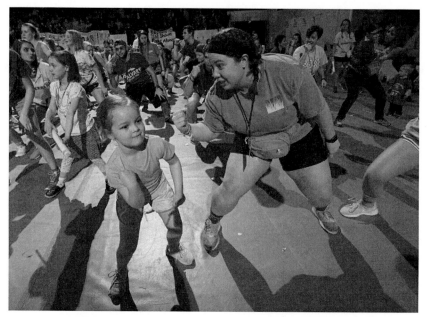

Young patients are welcome on the floor at DanceBlue

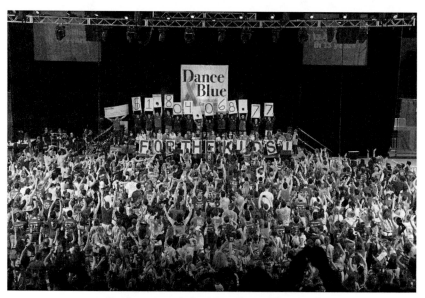

Students reveal the 2018 DanceBlue total

(Mark Cornelison/ UK Public Relations and Marketing)

49

To Be Continued

In late 2016, pediatric patients at the UK medical center, which now goes by the broader name "Kentucky Children's Hospital," were temporarily relocated to another section of the hospital so the acute care wing could be renovated.

The space would be redesigned not only to house updated equipment but also to make the place cheerier. Each pod of rooms would have its own distinct theme, such as rivers and streams, ocean life, or outer space.

The area was blocked off by drywall partitions, and for months, people could only wonder what was going on behind those temporary walls as they heard the sawing and hammering.

Five months after the construction project began, Jennifer was at the hospital preparing for a Joy Cart run. She noticed some of the barriers were down. The official reopening was just a couple weeks away. Curiosity got the best of her, and she walked down the halls of the section that had been closed off. The construction crews were gone for the evening, and the doors to each patient room were open.

It was all beautiful to her. Faux skylights brightened the space and drew attention to colorful murals over the nurses' stations. Even tiled patterns on the floor matched the themes.

She turned a corner into the "jungle pod." The walls were covered with paintings of monkeys swinging from vines and colorful parrots perched in trees. At the foot of each bed was a large lighted tile with an image that fit the theme—friendly-looking zebras, giraffes, and tiger cubs.

Jennifer approached the room in which Jarrett died.

"No, I'm not going in there," she told herself. "I need to keep walking . . . too many bad memories in there."

But it was as if a magnet pulled her eyes that way, and what she saw through the open door stopped her in her tracks. Pictured on the lighted panel at the end of the bed in that room was a large green tree frog. It reminded her of the one Granny Jeanne had accidentally killed back when Jarrett was small, just like the ones that had become a symbol of their affection for one another.

Jennifer's son and mother were both gone now, but this was a message to her.

"No one in that hospital or on the design team knew that story about the tree frog," Jennifer said. "There's no way that frog was purposely put there on our behalf."

There are no other frogs anywhere in the décor.

As The Joy Cart was approaching its 20th anniversary, Jennifer sometimes wondered if the project had run its course. It could be tiring to organize collections each week, shop for items, round up volunteers, and constantly seek funding. Was it still worth it?

Now she believed she had her answer.

The frog in the room where Jarrett drew his last breath was a message to her. She called it a "sledgehammer moment."

"It was Jarrett telling me I was supposed to be here—that I was doing exactly what I should be doing."

Each week, she is now happy to roll into that room and give a toy to a young patient.

She sees the frog and her heart jumps with joy.

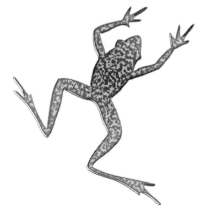

Afterword

Jarrett's Joy Cart still runs every Tuesday at Kentucky Children's Hospital, giving out two hundred and fifty toys per month. But it is so much more than a toy distribution project.

It supplies books, DVDs, and educational play items so patients with chronic illnesses can learn about their disease, and sponsors activities at an annual Childhood Cancer Survivors picnic. A $10,000 donation to the hospital made it possible to buy iPads, on mobile stations, that are loaded with interactive programs that explain medical procedures in ways children can understand.

Even now, long-time volunteer Guy Jones makes a ninety-minute drive to Lexington twice a month to help organize toys in the warehouse and deliver them in bins to the hospital. "I can't imagine not being there," he said. "I look forward to it each time. The whole project is blessed."

The Louisville Joy Cart still visits about thirty cancer patients every Thursday night at the facility, now renamed Norton Children's Hospital. It also provides lunch for the nurses there once a month.

It is largely funded by an annual spring gala at a country club, timed around the Kentucky Derby. Michael and Margaret Wagner's friends came up with that idea and put money and muscle behind it. The party seems to get bigger each year, with live music, good food, and an auction.

"I just don't see it stopping," Margaret said. "We've never had trouble getting donations or volunteers."

Two blocks away from Norton, there's a new cancer clinic. While children wait to see a doctor, they can pass the time in a room filled with toys – an area that bears the sign "Jarrett Mynear Pediatric Oncology Playroom."

Faithful volunteers continue to run the Seattle cart every other week, giving out about one hundred toys a month. Laurie Frink has been part of it from the beginning. She said she sees it as her mission to take the patients' minds off their sickness, even if just for a moment. "I'm not there to poke or prod," she said. "The biggest question I have for them is 'Do you want Hot Wheels or Legos?'"

Over the years, the Mynears have been contacted by people who want to start carts in Pennsylvania, Oregon, and Washington, as well as in Canada. There has been at least one toy delivery in China linked to the Kentucky project. Families and organizations are encouraged to embrace the mission of providing moments of joy to those who are struggling. However, the name "Jarrett's Joy Cart" is protected by copyright to ensure its 501(c)(3) non-profit status and integrity remain in compliance with federal and organizational guidelines.

There is no way to know how many endeavors have been inspired by Jarrett's Joy Cart or are in the works. E-mail suggests the number could be in the hundreds. Jarrett's story has been motivation for thousands of people looking for their own ways to carry out random acts of kindness.

There isn't a day that I don't think of Jarrett. I picture him now in Heaven, standing tall with a full head of wavy hair and two strong legs. He is out of pain and no doubt running around with all of the energy he built up and never got to use here on Earth. If God has a dog, Jarrett probably takes it for a walk every morning.

Jarrett's family asked me to sign an earlier version of this book to be buried with him. I felt honored and wrote simply:

Jarrett,
The best chapters of your story are yet to come. Take good notes and
we'll talk about it the next time we meet.
Your friend, Marvin

Acknowledgments

This book is the result of a lot of encouragement from a lot of people. First, I would like to thank Doug and Jennifer Mynear for their openness and patience with me as I conducted more than a hundred hours of interviews with them and their friends. It can't be easy to recount so many painful memories and be so honest about your emotions, yet they were always gracious.

Thanks to editor John Lynch for helping me round off the rough edges in my writing and to my friend K. J. Vigue II for lighting a fire under me to write a book in the first place. Susan Thurman can't be topped as a proofreader. My wife Elizabeth gives advice I trust the most.

The cover design is courtesy of talented graphic artist Creighton Matthews and some of the photos were taken by my good friend, Don Barker.

Above all, I have to thank Jarrett. It was impossible to have a negative attitude about anything when I was around him. His written story should help us all appreciate the millions of untold examples of courage and faith exhibited by cancer survivors. My own mother inspired those around her with the same upbeat outlook on life when she battled bone cancer. May we all recognize the angels among us.

Thank you, Jarrett, for showing us that it truly is more blessed to give than to receive.

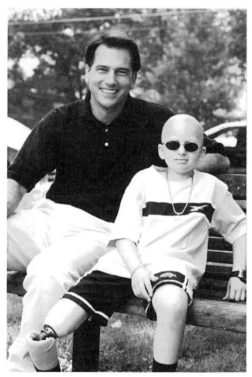

Marvin Bartlett and Jarrett Mynear, 2002

Links

Jarrett's Joy Cart
Postal address: *P.O. Box 24526, Lexington, KY 40524-2456*
Web address: *thejoycart.com*
Facebook: *facebook.com/Jarretts-Joy-Cart-Central-KY-112186148864151*

DanceBlue
Web address: *danceblue.org*
Facebook: *facebook.com/danceblue*
Twitter: *@UKDanceBlue*

Kentucky Children's Hospital
Postal address: *Fourth Floor, 800 Rose St., Lexington KY 40536*
Web address: *ukhealthcare.uky.edu/Kentucky-childrens-hospital*

The Dream Factory
Postal address: *410 W. Chestnut St., Suite 530, Louisville, KY 40202*
Web address: *dreamfactoryinc.org*

Kids Cancer Alliance
Web address: *kidscanceralliance.org*

To see and hear Jarrett in action, check out the playlists on the **Jarrett's Joy Cart YouTube channel.**

By purchasing this book, you have made a donation to ensure that Jarrett's Joy Cart continues to operate for years to come.